Mi'kmaq Puoinaq Two Spirit Medicine

Sexuality and Gender Variance, Spirituality and Culture

Dr Joseph Randolph Bowers

PhD Couns, MEd Couns., GCHE, CPNLP, BA Distinction, HACA

Foreward Contributor,

Elder Dr Daniel N. Paul

C.M., O.N.S., LLD, DLIT,

Ability Therapy Specialists Pty Ltd

Mi'kmaq Puoinaq Two Spirit Medicine

Sexuality and Gender Variance, Spirituality and Culture

Powerful medicine. A rare glimpse into sacred sexuality, gender, and identity. Honouring an often-hidden beautiful cultural landscape. Instructive, accessible, scholarly, relevant and practical. An insightful contribution to sexuality and gender, gay and lesbian, Native North American, and Indigenous studies. An integral textbook for courses in education, counselling, psychotherapy, psychology, social work, medicine, nursing, and health. Welcoming and empowering for youth, adults, and family. Dr Joseph Randolph Bowers is an Australian-Canadian Counsellor Psychotherapist and author of The Practice of Counselling, Sacred Teachings from the Medicine Lodge, and On the Threshold: Personal Transformation and Spiritual Awakening. Mi'kmaq Elder Dr Daniel N. Paul is a Canadian Historian and celebrated author of We Were Not the Savages: First Nations History. The authors reveal how Two Spirit and Traditional Medicine have always existed and are being rekindled in our times.

Keywords: Mi'kmaq, Micmac, First Nation, Two Spirit, Two-Spirits, Gay, Lesbian, Bisexual, Transgender, Intersex, Sexuality, Gender, Spirituality, Culture, Integral, Ecology, Native, North America, Traditional Medicine

Book Reviews

Speaking as a Mi'kmaq Mother and Grandmother and Aunt of many; and in my work in Counselling and Mental Health - this book is an exceptional resource that will help countless youth and adults with identity issues. This textbook is wholistic, deeply insightful, and practical. I wish we had this growing up and during my therapy training. We are happy to recommend the work of Dr Bowers and Elder Dr Paul.

- Bernice Doucette, Mi'kmaw Grandmother, Counsellor and Mental Health Practitioner, Eskasoni First Nation

Having known Dr Bowers for many years and during my former role as Editor of the Mi'kmaq Maliseet Nations News when he wrote the Eagle Medicine Column that later became his book *Sacred Teachings from the Medicine Lodge,* and as a Mi'kmaw woman and Aunt to many, I am delighted to suggest this book to anyone seeking information on Two Spirit, gender and sexuality issues. Like the work of Ruth Holmes Whitehead, Elder Dr Daniel N. Paul, and Professor Marie Battiste, this book may come to hold a special place among a rare collection of resources for our people to help youth and families, and as a textbook to inform counselling and health services. This book collects most work to date across an impressive spectrum, plus the authors honour traditional cultural values. The result is very unusual in the ways this book reflects and moves forward in cultural renewal and post-colonial healing.

- Wanda Duval-Muise, Mi'kmaq First Nation

Mi'kmaq Puoinaq Two Spirit Medicine: Sexuality and Gender Variance, Spirituality and Culture © 2019 Joseph Randolph Bowers, all rights reserved. Cover design © 2019 Joseph Randolph Bowers, all rights reserved. No part of this publication may be reproduced or transmitted in any form or by any means, electronic or mechanical, including photocopying, recording, or by any information retrieval and storage system, without prior written permission of the publisher.

Ability Therapy Specialists Pty Ltd | PO Box 4065, Armidale, New South Wales, Australia 2350 | E: abilitytherapyspecialists@gmail.com | W: www.abilitytherapyspecialists.com.au

Bibliographic Information: | Author: Bowers, Joseph Randolph. Foreward Author: Paul, Daniel N.. | Title: Mi'kmaq Puoinaq Two Spirit Medicine: Sexuality and Gender Variance, Spirituality and Culture
ISBN: 978-1-925034-10-3 [Paperback]
ISBN: 978-1-925034-08-0 [Hardcover]

Library of Congress Subject Headings: **Algonquian Indians**--Mi'kmaq; | **Indians of North America**--Canada--Eastern--Maritime Provinces, **Indians of North America**--Indian Philosophy--Medicine--Alternative Medicine--Psychology; **Indians of North America**--Religion, --Rites, Ceremonies; **Indians of North America**--Two-Spirits--Two-Spirit People--Indian men-women--Bardashes. | **Persons--Minorities--Sexual minorities**--Gays--Indian gays--Two Spirit people.

Keywords: Mi'kmaq, Micmac, First Nation, Two Spirit, Two-Spirits, Gay, Lesbian, Bisexual, Transgender, Intersex, Sexuality, Gender, Spirituality, Culture, Integral, Ecology, Native, North America, Traditional Medicine

Disclaimer: This book is produced for entertainment purposes only and is not an authoritative source of information. Readers ought to seek direct medical advice as your authoritative source of information. Under the limitations of the jurisdiction of NSW Australia the publisher disclaims all liability for all claims, expenses, losses, damages and costs any person may incur as a result of the information contained in this publication, for any reason, being inaccurate, or incomplete in any way or incapable or achieving any purpose. These statements do not disclaim statutory obligations as deemed necessary under the law.

Table of Contents

1	Title Page
2	About the Book
3	Book Reviews
4	Publication Data
5	Table of Contents
9	The Authors
10	Words from the Sacred Fire
11	Rocky Point Mi'kmaq Person, c. 1880
12	Acknowledgements
15	Dedication
16	Foreward Elder Dr Daniel N. Paul
	Going Deeper in Our Story
	About this Book
27	Preface
	Personal Empowerment
	Post-Colonial Contexts
	Culture & Spirituality
	Post-Colonial Spirituality
	Of Books & Medicine Bundles
44	Mi'kmaw Tli'suti – Mi'kmaq Language
	Puoinaq as Space for Vision
	Language and Cultural Revival
	Language is Culture, Ecology, Spirit
	Mi'kmaw Words Associated with Identity, Gender, Sexuality, and Two Spirit
61	Two Spirit Ethics

        Relations of Respect
        Relational Norms
        Incest Taboo and Child Protection
        Childhood and Identity Formation
        Internet and Social Media
        Adult Survivors of Sexual Abuse
        Early Adult Initiation
        Drawing Firm Lines in the Sand
        Learning Our Ways, Unlearning Colonial Ways

78   Gender Identity, Gender Variance
        Analysis of Western Cultures
        Mi'kmaq History and Early Colonial Contexts
        Colonial Gender and Sexuality
        Colonial Gendered Relations
        19th Century Mi'kmaq and the Victorian Gender Paradox
        Two Spirit Contexts
        Stigma as Waning Moon
        Youth Suicide

105   Two Spirit Ways of Knowing
        Indigenous Standpoint
        Cultural Traditions
        The Kluskap Cycles
        The Switch Dance
        From Confusion to Sacred Ecology

122   Two Spirit Ceremony as Life
        Trauma and Healing Methods
        Death as Passage and Growth
        Medicine Sacred Circle as Science and Life
        Mi'kmaq Wholistic Ecological Model

139   Puoinaq Cultural Reawakening
        Visions of Mi'kmaw Research-as-Ceremony
        Challenges Ahead
        Mi'kmaw Oral Tradition
        Body-based Memory
        Decolonising the Sacred Sexual
        Mi'kmaw Cosmology

157 Two Spirit Medicine Teachings
        Initiation Ceremonies
        Men's and Women's Medicine
        Two Spirit Service and Skill
        Two Spirit Purpose and Vocation
        Depression - This Too Will Pass
        True Nature, True Identity

171 Two Spirit Oral Tradition
        The Wigwam of Family
        The Sacred Pipe of Family
        The Meaning of Traditional

182 Ambassadors of Memory
        Looking Back, Looking Forward
        From Plausible to Instructive
        Ancestral Memory and Recovery

193 Two Spirit Gender Deconstruction
        Song Lines and Medicine Trails
        M'sit No'kama - All My Relations
        Story as Medicine

203 A Tale of Two Spirits
        Ta'pu Miijaqamijjk Puoinaq Paq'tism
        Wanderer
        Waking Up
        Rising Up on Wings
        Raven's Two Eyed Seeing
        Paq'tism Arising
        Paq'tism Awakening
        Surrender… Please…
        Shadow as Passage to Life
        Embracing Shadows
        Two Spirits Becoming Whole
        Post-Trauma Recovery
        Sa'qawei Paq'tism Speaks

218 Two Spirit Narrative of Origins
        Kepmitelsi Two Spirit Pride

　　　　　Ancient Old Ones - Two Spirit Beings
　　　　　Conference of the Four Winds
　　　　　The Two Spirit Vision
　　　　　Ancient Grandmother Turtle Pipe
　　　　　Two Spirit Healing of Nations
　　　　　Teaching the First Mi'kmaq
　　　　　Prophesies of the Great Suffering
　　　　　The First Two Spirit Mi'kmaq
　　　　　The Great Suffering
　　　　　A World for our Children
　　　　　Visions of Hope

236　　Bibliography

250　　The Publisher

The Authors

Dr Joseph Randolph Bowers PhD Couns, MEd Couns, GCHC, CPNLP, BA Distinction, HACA, is a Senior Counsellor Psychotherapist and Behaviour Specialist. He taught for two decades at Australian and Canadian universities in Counselling, Education, and Indigenous Studies. His works are kept in special collections with the Mi'kmaq Resource Centre, Cape Breton University, and Tepi'ketuek Mi'kmaq Archives, University of Saskatchewan. Since 2007, he is an Associate Scholar with the Centre for World Indigenous Studies USA. He is an author of over two hundred publications, including books *The Practice of Counselling, Sacred Teachings from the Medicine Lodge,* and *On the Threshold: Personal Transformation and Spiritual Awakening*. Dr Bowers works in community practice with Ability Therapy Specialists Pty Ltd in the mountains of New South Wales Australia.

Mi'kmaq Elder Dr Daniel N. Paul C.M., O.N.S., LLD, DLIT, is an historian and the celebrated author of *We Were Not the Savages: First Nations History*. His most recent book *Chief Lightning Bolt* is an inspired novel set in pre-contact Mi'kmaq society. Among many awards, Elder Paul received an Honorary Doctor of Letters from Université Sainte-Anne (1997), Honorary Doctor of Law from Dalhousie University (2013), Order of Canada (2005), Order of Nova Scotia (2002), and the esteemed Grand Chief Donald Marshall Memorial Elder Award (2007). Elders Daniel and Patricia live in Halifax and enjoy life with many grand and great-grandchildren.

Words from the Sacred Fire

Epse'n sisvey nkamhamun, pana'tu wjipenukewey ka'qn

- Enter my heart sacred fire, open Eastern door

Nukumij npisuney tumaqn, Sekewa' skituknukewey tepknuset

- Grandmother Pipe Medicine, Rise Western Moon

Sa'qawey npisuni nkijj, Ketapekiweuksiek aq alasutmelsewuksiek

- Ancient Mother Medicine, Singing for us, praying for us

Iknemuin napukwetunen tel koqajeimk

- Give our lives to your work

Editor's Note: Lovingly translated during 2007, by Elder Katherine Sorbey from the western door of Mi'kma'ki residing in eastern Quebec.

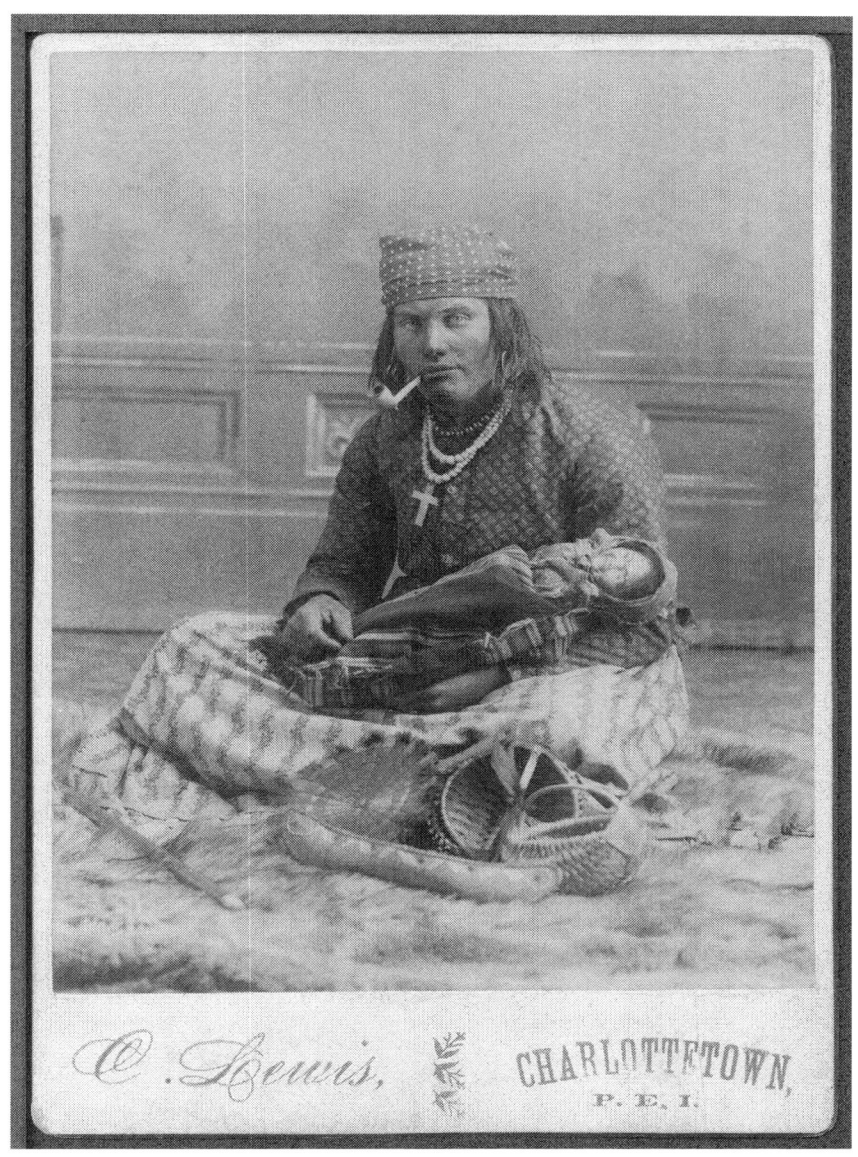

Rocky Point Mi'kmaq Person, c. 1880

Editor's Note: See under 'Gender Identity, Gender Variance' for permissions and in-depth discussion of this photograph of an unnamed Rocky Point Mi'kmaq person, taken between 1880 and 1920.

Acknowledgements

Wela'lioq, thank you, to elders who prodded and inspired me to write about Two Spirit ways.

Elder Muin'skw of Whycobah First Nation.

Friends and family at Eskasoni First Nation.

Elder Chief Frank Meuse, friends and family of Bear River First Nation.

Elder Jamie Jermey, friends and family of Acadia First Nation, and Wildcat Reservation, Wela'lin.

Elder Todd Labrador AKA Amalkat Sam'qwanijtuk – One Who Dances on Water, Wela'lin.

Elder Ellen Hunt, French Acadian and Mi'kmaq friends and family who gather each summer in the meeting grounds of our Ancestors at La'Have. Wela'lioq.

Sister Ruth Holmes Whitehead for taking time out of your retirement. Your knowledge and insight are invaluable and continue to guide our work.

Elder Dr Daniel Paul, Danny, for continual inspiration and kind words. Thank you for friendship while at Cape Breton University. Thank you for agreeing to write the Foreward and all that this means to me and to so many others. Truly a gift of kindness.

Elder Professor Marie Battiste for your beautiful kinship welcome and support in work and life. Wela'lin nitap.

Elder Georgina Doucette, Ruby and Kyle (Becca) for your incredible hospitality and taking us into your home; and dear sisters Bernice and children, the late Jenny and children, and good brothers Vaughan, Mike, Noel Jr. (Seymour), Daniel, Donald and John, and all our family at Eskasoni First Nation. Wela'lioq.

Elder gkisedtanamoogk for guidance and teachings around the Sacred Fire, and spiritual wisdom.

Elders Albert and Murdina Marshall of Eskasoni, for inspiring teachings and witness to life and hope. Murdina the world misses you dearly.

Elders of Eskasoni First Nation for welcome into the Wigwam of the Elders to tend Sacred Fire during the Elder's Healing Retreats.

To colleagues at the Mi'kmaq Resource Centre, Cape Breton University, especially Diane Chisholm. To faculty and staff at Cape Breton University School of Education, particularly Susan Basso, Terry MacDonald, Diane Janes, Maureen Finlayson, Patrick Howard, Jane Lewis, Coleen Moore-Hayes, and Catherine O'Brien.

John Boylan and colleagues at the Public Archives and Records Office of Prince Edward Island, Public Services Archivist.

Professors John Sumarah, Jacques Goulet, and the late Jim Foster and of course Redge Craig.

Professor Victor Minichello, and Professor David Plummer - thank you.

Elder Steve Widders for welcome to country.

Elder Aunty Pat Dixson for welcome to country, you are dearly missed.

Elder Aunty Diane Roberts, for the reconnect of heart and life with our people.

Elder Raelene Councillor for kinship welcome and drawing me into your beautiful Broome and WA family.

Sister Morning Star Annette LeBlanc-Power for traveling with, for many years.

Dr Dwayne Andrew Kennedy, for ancient friendship.

Elders Grace and John. Jonna and Chris, and children. Donna and Daniel and kids. Lisa and Dennis, and kin. Kay and David, and all the mob.

Elders Jeanette and Joseph. Angela, Erica, Kyle, and kin.

Joe Bergeron, brother and friend.

Gloria Wood, keep exploring the Great Oneness.

Mi'kmaq Elders who gifted the name Kisiku Sa'qawei Paq'tism so long ago…

Catherine-Ann Fuller, see you in the snowflakes.

Tuma Young and Nick Honig, and the Wabanaki Two-Spirit Alliance, Wela'lioq.

Michael Weir. 'Just wait and see.'

Bernice Doucette and Wanda Duval-Muise, for reading the manuscript and writing reviews. Heartfelt thanks in encouraging support.

Seventh generation. Younger Elders, this book is for you.

Dedication:

For all readers and seekers on the way.

May these words speak to your heart and give insight, hope, and encouragement.

Take only what is useful to you personally, and seriously, disregard the rest.

Please pass on this book to someone you feel might benefit from support and encouragement or a new way of seeing, feeling, and thinking.

But like all things in life, this book is not for everyone and is certainly not for the faint of heart.

In whatever way you choose to believe, may strength and wisdom of heart be your medicine always.

M'sit No'kama, Ta'ho.

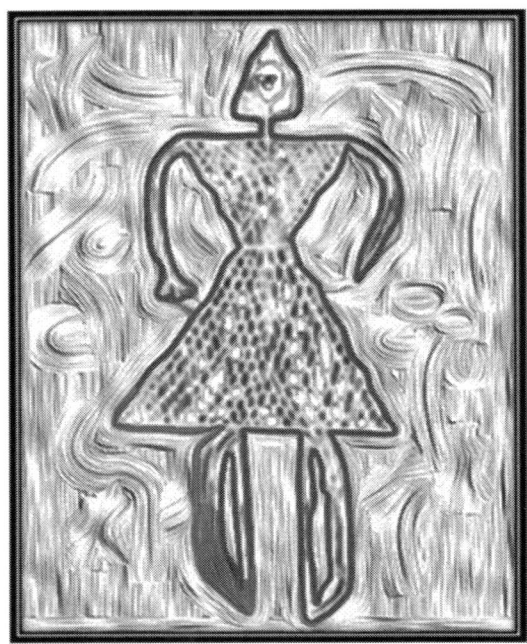

Foreward Elder Dr Daniel N. Paul

Over the ages many humans, as they moved toward what they perceived to be civilized behaviour, actually moved away from toleration of the differences of others toward intolerance. Many factors were involved in this transition.

However, the development of religious creeds that rejected tolerance and promoted greed for personal enrichment were one of the primary sources of this movement toward the darker side of human development. Horrors such as brutal discrimination because of race, gender, and sexual orientation, among many other forms of identity held up as targets for violence, were the evils that sprang up from this type of developing mind-set.

As history relates, Europeans in particular were more industrious at developing modes of hatred for the differences of others. Under the guise of spreading what they deemed 'civilisation' and 'Christianity' they destroyed or badly damaged the civilisations of the Americas, Australia,

Africa, and Asia. History shows how they honed and tested their intolerance and inclinations upon each other and the other.

Religious wars raged for centuries among European nations. The thirst among the continent's leadership for tools of war to amass great riches and power became insatiable. The most horrific result of this rests with weapons of mass destruction that are fully capable of exterminating all humanity and all other living creations that Great Spirit endowed upon Mother Earth.

Perhaps racial hatred based upon a person's skin colour or racial origins was the worst product of European intolerance. Over the past five decades discrimination based on race, gender, and sexual orientation has abated considerably. However, there is still a very long way to go. Plenty of religious leaders still rail against one another's beliefs and condemn those who don't adhere to their views and teachings. But there are also many among them who now preach conciliation, tolerance, and peace.

Today, the most discriminated against group of people are women of the developing world and those whose sexual orientation is not viewed as 'straight' or 'normal' by their country's religious and political leaders. In many countries, women cannot even drive cars and can be killed by stoning for adultery and so on. Homosexual orientation in many of the same countries is considered a capital offence.

Much of this status quo can be chalked up to ignorance of what people see as the unknown. When people become knowledgeable, they see they have nothing to fear. In the same way, when you learn about people of any given nation or gender who are not heterosexual but have the same basic desires for companionship and sexual relations with members of their own sex, you begin to realise that the extended histories of intolerance are largely based in fear of the unknown. Ironically these individuals with same sex attraction have been systematically ostracized for centuries by many so-called civilised cultures.

Ignorance is the root cause of this situation. If people who are indeed ignorant would take the time to inquire and educate themselves about the people that they debase blindly they would find the self-same aspirations, hopes, and fears common to all people and quite close to home. We are not that different from each other. But ironic that gender and sexual difference is one of the defining themes of our era simply because globally very many cultures now awaken to attitudes of tolerance and knowledge-based support of same-gender love and relationships.

Dr Bowers suggests, 'It is important to remember that we are all deeply relational creatures who need authentic, honest, and open communication. To share our inner world with each other is actually an incredibly complicated process with all kinds of mishaps and blocks that can prevent transparent and helpful experiences of intimacy. In this context my use of intimacy does not mean sexualised energy. Quite the contrary. Healthy human intimacy has very little to do with sexual energy. At the best of times adults find it often challenging to share their inner world with each other. Add the inherent pressures of childhood growth and development combined with the youthful emergence of independence, and you have a situation that takes a great deal of patience, insight, and genuine loving concern.'

In Two Spirit Medicine you will find exploration of this intimate knowledge of humanity's heart and soul – something we all share. Something common to our family and nation. You will be challenged to listen and feel your own trials and tribulations by coming to terms with the life stories and experiences of non-heterosexual people living within a largely heterosexual world. In the process, this reflective scholarly and deeply traditional inquiry may surprise you, inspire and educate you, and become a powerful companion for you on your path and work in life. Allow me now to address the theme of tolerance from perspectives that may assist the reader in appreciating the nature of this book and the topics offered here.

Going Deeper in Our Story

It is a pleasure to offer introduction to Two Spirit Medicine written by Dr Joseph Randolph Bowers. I call him Randy. Allow me to begin with a bit of history.

When I was born a Registered Indian in 1938 on Shubenacadie Indian Reserve in Nova Scotia, I was not considered a Canadian British Subject. I was a Ward of the Crown. As Wards of the Crown we had no civil and human rights in this country.

We were not permitted to vote in elections, we could be legally barred by law from public places such as pool rooms without cause, it was illegal for us to buy a case of beer, and so on, and most tellingly, we had very little recourse to law. In contractual arrangements, we had the same legal status as drunks and insane persons.

I speak from experience. Federal Indian Agents had God like powers over us, they controlled our lives from the cradle to the grave. And, most of them thought themselves to be our betters. This brings to mind an amusing story. I was a rebel against a racially intolerant system since I was very young and was not intimidated by Indian Agent authority.

During a discussion with an Indian Agent in the late 1950s, I dared to disagree with him. He commented: 'You're not very respectful of your betters!' In response I said, 'The reason that you perceive such is that you assume that I've met my betters, which I haven't, and I won't until the day I die and meet my Maker, then I will concede that I've met my betters!' He was flabbergasted and left my company not a happy camper.

Up until 1961 I worked at many trades and support positions, carpenter, labourer, harvester, factory worker, and many others that are far too numerous to mention here. When I got into management in 1961, I remembered well the vital importance of supporting people, and treating them with fairness and respect. Such fair treatment is a must to have a successful existence, treat other humans with the utmost tolerance and respect, and give them human dignity, and most will respond in kind.

We, and our ancestors, have been victimized by intolerance for centuries. You might like to read about this history in my book We Were Not the Savages, that details the colonial relations over the past five hundred years.

Racism towards us, although not as blatant as it used to be, is still displayed openly in Nova Scotia. For instance, in Cornwallis Park there was a statue of British Colonial Governor Edward Cornwallis, a man who decided in 1749 to try to exterminate the Mi'kmaq on Peninsula Nova Scotia. After concerted efforts during January 2018, the statue was removed and placed in storage. However, the Mi'kmaq-colonial encounter is not widely understood.

It took a long time for Registered Indians to make some progress in acquiring a measure of civil and human rights in this country, attitudes are slowly changing, but we still have a long way to go. However, happily, intolerance has been publicly and forcefully addressed to some degree over the last few decades by some very notable people. Michael Levine (2011), in *Lessons at the Halfway Point*, says, 'If you don't personally get to know people from other racial, religious or cultural groups, it's very easy to believe ugly things about them and make them frightening in your mind.' Levine's advice would, if followed around the world, reduce conflicts among humans significantly.

Many things are changed by intolerance. The way people feel able to gain employment, seek assistance from professionals, move freely or not about the world, access food, health care, medicine, and education. The way we learn by experience in society, and how we resolve problems as they arise. For example, we might seek a trades person when dealing with a leaking roof or have someone in our family lucky enough to have studied building or carpentry.

The ways we get by and make life better for self and family make for the paths and resources that end up part of our upbringing. Native people in Canada have had lack of access. This is the fundamental issue of racism and systemic violence that prevents us getting by, getting an education, and having more choice and control of how we engage in society. I speak from experience. You might look at my titles and see the accomplishments. This was not always the case.

On June 13, 2011, I received an Honorary Diploma from Halifax's Nova Scotia Community College Institute of Technology. This was an important acknowledgment. In some ways Randy's tome on Two Spirit issues relates to similar treatment that is accorded to Two Spirit People that is rooted in intolerance! However, you slice this word intolerance, you get the same result - people do not work together for mutual benefit. People divide themselves from others. People might think they are better than you, but this is illusion. Randy calls this projecting. This is true. You project like a movie camera on the screen something that is inside of you. This means that prejudice says more about you than the person you project onto. In fact, that person receiving your projection needs to discover who they are apart from your projecting onto them. The barriers this creates between people are many. The result is social isolation. To isolate means to separate equals. This dynamic is harmful to everyone. But consider the power of the word that means we are equals become separated, isolated.

I have seen this dynamic throughout history. We can read about this in the letters of British colonial leaders, some of who are still upheld in Canada as founders of cities, provinces, or the country. The history is actually extremely clear. Those who read the evidence now acknowledge the racism and violence for what that is and was, even in the context of the times. Historians in past covered over or sidestepped this truth to save face or deny the truth for the sake of political trends. But when you look clearly at intolerance the truths of history are plain and simple.

People do not act in a vacuum. People act in the ways they act. We are loving and kind to others, or we are confused, intolerant, and even abusive. People have to find inwardly the choice to make good attitudes. If you do not question what you receive as a child, and continue to not ask questions as an adult, you may find yourself acting in ways that are unkind to others. This may not come to your awareness because you are too busy projecting onto others the lies you have learned.

Long before receiving the Honorary Diploma I was a student at the same school in early 1970. At the time I recognised a need for a high school Diploma to make career progress. I studied for and wrote my GED exams, consequently acquiring a High School Diploma. This was an acquisition that has been a tremendous help in achieving career and life goals.

Randy once told me the story of his father who had a similar experience. He was the eldest of eight so left school very early to work and support the family with needed income. Like me much of Joe Bowers time was spent studying for qualifications at night time after a busy day at work. We do what we have to do sometimes to get ahead for the sake of our families.

About this Book

In this book that you will read, Randy shares many different perspectives and insights about the Two Spirit experience. There is something here for most people. From my perspective, the common threads around intolerance make Two Spirit issues very simple and direct. No human being deserves projection of prejudice or any kind of projection at all. This way people objectify others causes harm. Harm in history or harm now, both lead to poor outcomes.

Society and family life are best based on tolerance and respect, honour and shared mutual truth. To find the latter you need the former. You cannot build a relationship without tolerance and respect. This is true in a marriage as much as in a business or social project.

From my perspective as a student of history, there are points of evidence in other North American contexts where documentations can easily be viewed as pointing to the Two Spirit gender variant experience. Letters or writings of missionaries, legal documents, or other evidence points to this phenomenon. Randy asked me whether I found this evidence while researching Mi'kmaw history. My response was not yet, but I was not looking for this either. The interesting point was that when future generations of scholarship read the data and search for what might have been overlooked, evidence may come forward. But that is a work for the future.

If, however, from an historical and sociological view, we ask if there was a likelihood of Two Spirit gender variance in Mi'kmaw culture the more realistic answer leans toward yes. Yes, it is likely that this phenomenon existed in past. It may have been called different things. Randy explores some of this territory in this book, so it is not my place here to discuss further. The point I would like to make is that there is more likelihood than we might first suspect, especially in my generation.

The younger generation may take a view different from we older folks. They may see what they see in their culture or experience as reflected in history. This has a layer of our projecting onto history what we want to see, but also when we question this in realistic ways, history is always a blend of the truth that exists and the truth that we want to see or don't want to see. The key is getting the mix right and actually taking a balanced view. They call this historiography. This is a field that studies the decisions and reasons for how history is written, discussed, and co-created in each generation. We native people need to take part in this discussion and to influence outcomes that provide for our unique perspectives on history.

When it comes to Two Spirit or what are the elements of this, we see gender differences and we see sexuality differences. We know from sociology these happen across all cultures around the world. In most cases, Indigenous cultures are more open to variations than cultures dominated by religions or over-arching philosophies.

Indigenous cultures tend to take a more inherent view of human experience. In other words, we allow what emerges in personal experience and nature. The point is not to control and dominate nature and self, but to nurture a relation of respect with what is real and what is happening in nature.

As soon as we stray from this path, we get in trouble. The old stories of our Elders say this in many different ways. When you read some of the ethnographies by Ruth Holmes Whitehead, who was also in touch with Randy about this book and Two Spirit issues, we begin to understand that Mi'kmaw teachers were oriented to help young people take on and reflect upon values that build personal agency, personal power, and to act with honour and respect.

Even sacred ceremonies and very sacred traditions have this element of teaching the better way to live, and the ways we can deal with crisis or personal doubt. The practices point to basic social and emotional values that help youth and adults address problems and move forward with honour and respect.

From our current views across science and historiography we know that there are many issues covered over by the values of people who wrote the histories. We know for example how this effected women's rights in European cultures around the world. We can re-read the history and in certain times and places there may not be any mention of women beyond their legal or economic value and status. It may read like counting sheep or cattle. Arguments may arise between men who fight to own a woman. During whole periods of European history this may be the case, and women's writing that survived may remain rare and precious.

In an even more pervasive way, Two Spirit experience was not written into history, or more precisely was white washed out of history by people who could not reflect on the beauty and diversity of humanity. One reason was that European cultures objectified women's status to such a degree that gender roles were extremely male-dominated and rigid. Much fear and projection were associated with anything outside the culture's norms of gender and sexuality. Much of this had been for centuries dictated by the church and social systems that had grown up to have enormous power over people's everyday lives.

Prior to colonial contact, such a vast machine of social disorder and oppression did not exist for native cultures in North America. Psychologists actually call the social condition of disorder and oppression a form of mass psychosis or macro psychosocial disorder. Sociologists with psychological training examine culture-wide trends for signs of degradation into oppressive regimes, and a global scale and nation-based scoring system is commonly used today that provides countries with more objective measures for social wellness verses social disorder. Therefore, it is not that far-fetched to look at colonial histories and actually quite fairly and objectively assess the status quo in social relations.

Native nations during the early days of colonial relations had no comparison and no idea how extensive this social disorder was until it was too late. We have studied and observed this now for 500 years, so our take on things is fairly realistic and objective. Our objectivity is partly based on our philosophy of detachment in support of creation. What is remains what is, regardless our desire for change. A basic attitude of acceptance underpins native culture because we seek to remain in harmony with nature. This does not mean we do not have a warrior tradition. But even here, native warrior traditions are spiritually grounded in principles of honour, respect, truth, humility, listening, learning, and justice. Our values tend to balance the process of engaging with conflict.

For the Mi'kmaw people colonisation quickly enough moved past relations of apparent respect and honour into relations based on greed, control of land and water resources, and oppressive ownership of everything to such a degree that freedom was lost for everyone including European settlers and their children. But by then the wave of immigration and domination was well underway. The Americas were never quite the same again.

When you consider these points of view, you quickly realise that Two Spirit gender and sexuality diversity likely existed among the Mi'kmaq as something honourable and normal, just as women's leadership and inherent value was highly respected among our people. But you may not find direct and clear written evidence of either of these points depending on where you look and who was doing the writing.

The point about medicine traditions is interesting. There are many perspectives on this today. Most discussions can easily lead to arguments of belief. But the point is that this may always have been the case. We know that there were medicine keepers, wise women, wise men, solitary individuals, people who studied herbal lore and kept a store of medicines. We know that there were others who specialised in crafts, practical skills, hunting, or gathering. There were those who carried knowledge of the seasons. Again, a degree of everyday caution rests around medicine keepers because in one sense their knowledge of herbal lore or spirituality was different from other people. What you don't know may arise fear, so you are weary until you trust a person with powers of knowledge. This is a natural human process and speaks to the trusted place that medicine keepers held within the culture.

As other examples, we know from historical evidence that our people were experts on mapping the stars, that they were good at ocean passage for fishing, and that tracking in the deep woods of this region demanded very good survival skills. There is so much we have lost. It is not farfetched to imagine that we have lost a small minority of individuals whose specialisation included gender variance and sexuality diversity some of whom were medicine keepers. It is not far-fetched to imagine some of these people having same-sex relationships or marriages. It is not far-fetched to imagine certain individuals attaining a high degree in the arts of their choosing, and we can look around today and find people who dedicate their life to similar pursuits. The Puoinaq medicine tradition is not lost but being reawakened in our times. Two Spirit movements are an expression of this wider cultural healing.

These situations of same sex relationships may exist today and where the adults involved are honest, honourable, and respectful, family and community get used to things and tolerate or accept people for who they are. This is the native way more or less. To see this in history is plausible. To see this in Mi'kmaw history is even more plausible given the core of native values are generally tolerant and accepting of diversity in creation and in people.

A few years back Randy published a paper on the nature of diversity in creation and how native cultures provide more space for acceptance and tolerance (Bowers 2007c). This is not a new area for contemporary studies. But what is new here is the combination of studies that allow people today to challenge old prejudices and to move forward with supportive relations in society.

Today we see this lack of tolerance still around same-sex marriages, raising of children by same-sex couples, and generally allowing and helping these minorities to get on with life in society. It is not that we have to do extra work here. It is just that like my early days, people in society need to have a positive attitude. People need to have space and time to help one another. People need to be able to apply for a job or school diploma or GED or degree, and not be rejected because of their colour, beliefs, who they sleep with, or who they call their partner or spouse.

In conclusion, I encourage you to be tolerant and forgiving towards your human brothers and sisters. When you view your co-workers and others do not let race, colour, religion, sexual orientation, etc., demean him/her in your eyes. Instead see him/her as an equal, and always treat fellow humans with dignity and respect. Your reward will be a happy and prosperous lifetime.

- Elder Dr Daniel N. Paul, 10 January 2019, Mi'kma'ki

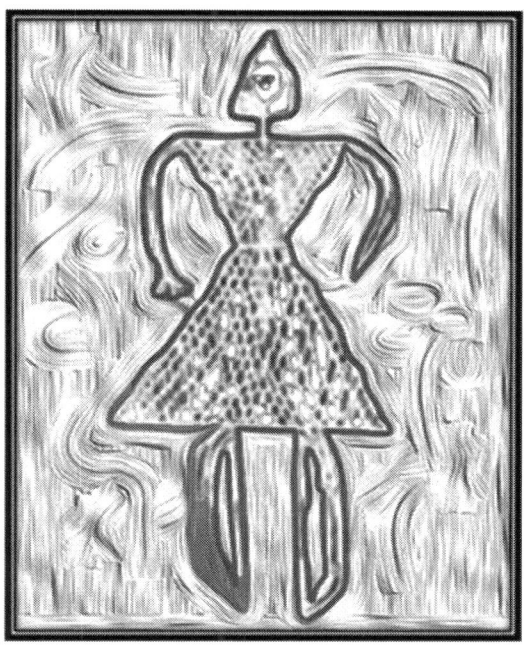

Preface

Pjila'si – Welcome, come in, sit down by the sacred fire. Elders in We'koqma'q - Waybobah, Eskisoqnik - Eskasoni, L'setkuk - Bear River or Muin Sipi, Wildcat and Malikiaq - Acadia, and other places asked me independently and at different times to please write a book about Two Spirit. 'We need this. Our youth need this.' That was well over 10 years ago.

There is actually a lot more information out there now. If you look for websites and Facebook pages or groups, you will find helpful resources. Today we also have greater acknowledgement of diversity in native identities. Sexual health has moved forward generally and in Indigenous contexts as well. There are new generations of Aboriginal teachers and scholars nowadays, and the efforts of national and international Indigenous movements are showing meaningful though limited results. These include the Centre for World Indigenous Studies based in the USA. Our affiliation with CWIS for over ten years has opened opportunities for progress in Indigenous education and advocacy.

Modern scholarship across the fields of counselling, sociology, health, and education, as well as Indigenous studies over the past twenty years rely heavily on deconstructing prior models of learning and research. This work has led to widespread support for making both tasks more honest. To these ends, there are many tools that have emerged to help keep on track our various sources of information, curriculum, research, and professional practice.

There are for example approaches like the use of personal narrative and story within professional discourse. In the therapy fields where most of my daily work happens these methods are highly valued. In research, it is now common practice to intentionally reveal one's identity and purpose in writing, giving readers and other researchers a clearer reflection on the contexts that defines a work. We have standpoint theory, a very helpful construct in identity research, gay and lesbian studies, and Indigenous studies. This theory suggests that every writing has a standpoint, even and especially work that hides its origins and values. In fact, the present-day approaches across many fields aligns with the idea that hidden knowledge constitutes efforts to maintain power relations, as power is exercised often more by hiding and controlling access to information.

Then there are methods in education that have long standing value and are quite helpful. Like the pedagogy of the oppressed arising from Latin America and Freire's work (1978), which provides many tools like analysis, critique, comparison, contrast, strategic use of sacred or mundane texts and media, mobilisation, strategic social action, protest, resistance, and finding sources of inner and social resilience.

From Australia we are given educaring methods that combine the Indigenous ethics of loving kindness and justice-making with the intentional translation of Aboriginal family and community practices into the classroom and research halls of learning. Educaring methods gleaned from Professor Judy Atkinson's (2006) work combines with notions of Indigenous sacred traditions, where these intersect with modern forms of information exchange and learning.

For example, within Aboriginal Song Lines and Dreaming practices there are very many teachings that arise which over the colonial history and within the invader-mentality are side-tracked and diminished. These forms of traditional knowledge are re-tracked back to origins, as it were, and given credibility by acknowledgement practices that include personal healing, loss and grief work, creative agency and craft-as-transformational, and therapeutic reconnecting-work with our ancestral and genetic memories.

From Canada the global community is given much wisdom in post-colonial reflections and methods across all fields of practice, and in community-based work, and family life education. Post-colonial methods are championed by Professor Marie Battiste (2004) whose Mi'kmaq identity deepens the relevance of these approaches within this book and the life-work this represents for so many of us. Marie is so highly respected and valued internationally. We have seen this in many countries and felt a deep pride in her as kin. Post-colonial efforts have become such a large field of practice that it is difficult to summarise.

The key features that we highlight for you relate to how we use the method in daily work and in research-as-life and life-as-research. To engage the 'post' means to use another perspective other than the obvious observation of whatever meets your focus. The method requires you to observe with your eyes and ears, but also to take another view or feeling. This experience is valuable in all manners, especially in therapy where people seek new points of view. The 'post' is also about a socio-political shift away from certain values and beliefs towards more resourceful attitudes and principles.

For example, how we value women's role and place within society constitutes a 'post' after of colonial experience. The 'post' in this sense can be about recovery from the trauma, violence, or limited perspectives of the colonial mindset. In this way, 'post' is acknowledging that there are different mindsets to begin with, and that everyone exercises their views in symbolic and behavioural ways, so that it is healthier and more productive to acknowledge your standpoint and co-create ways of thinking and acting that build mutuality.

The 'colonial' of post-colonial highlights that history and values intersect, not only in past but right now, in this time. Colonial beliefs and practices can be found in present day ideas, systems of governance, education curriculums, ways of leadership or following leaders, approaches to community life, family, and in the ways that people define their identity. A wide range of values have been identified and can be more easily 'picked out' when you use this set of skills. This provides everyone with a different landscape of choices and response-options, when we come to terms with what were in colonial cultures the hidden terms of engagement.

From many international sources we are given gay and lesbian histories of emancipation dating back into the 19th century and earlier. From these arise modern expressions of feminism, gender studies, queer theory, and transgender discourse. Around these rather sacred fires of learning and social agency gather a wide range of practices and methods in teaching, learning, research, and professional methods. These approaches provide a collectively powerful deconstructive edge, but also and more so, the basis for creative reconstruction of culture and new forms of status-quo that are continually transformed inside the fires of personal power.

Personal Empowerment

How important to realise that all knowledge is actually between your ears and no theory or idea can live on a page or in electronic systems. There must be a form of intelligence that guides knowledge, even within cyberspace artificial intelligence requires a form of agency.

Native people traditionally know that personal power rests in the heart without writing the words, because knowledge is oral and based in personal encounter and communication. But nowadays youth are expected to perform in schools that not only seek to provide native systems of knowledge but also bi-cultural literacy. The expectations for native youth to succeed in the current climate are enormous. For LGBTIQ and Two Spirit youth we can easily add to these typical pressures in growing up issues around the social impacts and internalisation of racism, homophobia, and heteronormative values.

This is why, when Elder Daniel Paul offered in kindness a foreword for this book, his gift of belief in my work completely blew me away. It has meant so much to me, I cannot begin to express. Elder Danny's writing was so powerful his words had to begin this book. In respect for his gift I asked him would he like his name on the book cover? He agreed. This gesture is huge on his part. Not only in respect for my work but for the Mi'kmaw youth that Danny wished to reach with his message of tolerance, kindness, and love.

Danny understands the range of pressures that native youth face in today's world. In many ways the issues are similar to past generations, but with a contemporary social media twist. There are other ways that the structures of society, more broadly, and Mi'kmaq society have moved forward and changed. In many ways the world today is more complex, given to higher degrees of laws, rules, codes, structures, and it can seem like everything is so well defined that there is no space for youth to grow into creating visions for tomorrow.

As only one example, today there are more fences everywhere. Land use terms have evolved and continue to change. Though native people have lived with land and water use restrictions for many generations, there are increasing pressures on these natural systems from all sides. Including the higher degree of actual use of natural resources by native communities, i.e. through having built homes, businesses, and facilities. Youth may find it harder generally to forage, enjoy nature, and learn the traditional ways of ecology that were at one time common to all peoples of the planet. The incremental changes over time as well as current fast paced change generate new social and ecological relationships and contexts. These situations create new problems for youth in terms of mental, emotional, physical, and spiritual health. Often such problems may not surface until the mid-teen years when identity formation and innate needs for initiation into adulthood kicks in, giving rise to conflicts within the soul of youth.

Perhaps we might say, prepare yourself. This book holds little back. Depending on your values, beliefs, and cultural perspectives this book may challenge, inspire, or affirm. We remind, in native ways nothing is unclean.

Yes, there are many areas that are taboo, and many other areas that should remain taboo. But this book is all about respect and finding our way. What was perhaps taboo in another generation is here part of respectful relations. This concept of historical development is key to understanding how this book came to be.

In these pages we will openly discuss Two Spirit and GLBTIQ+ issues, gender and sexuality, spirituality and culture, religion and colonialism, western cultural values and western religion. There are few stones we do not overturn to see what lies beneath the assumptions we all have grown up with over the years. All this is done with utmost respect and to accomplish this also takes many years of reflection. To say things in the best way possible requires time to brew.

At the same time sometimes saying things is never easy or neat and tidy. This book is really about asking the hard questions. But more so, the purpose of doing this work is to raise the Sacred Fires of Hope, to remember the Sunrise Ceremony of our Elders. To provide youth with a way forward in dialogue with our Elders. This is really why the Two Spirit narrative is so important – not for us but for our nation. Not just for our nation, but for all nations. By recovery of identity and personhood, we show a path of regenerative human ecology that is needed now among all peoples of earth.

In retrospect, regeneration is not really complete without regression and healing, without facing head on and in personal ways the violence of colonialism that sadly includes religious bias, prejudice and fear. For native people, for those of minority status, for the poor and dispossessed, for the elderly and forgotten, there are so many ways that contemporary cultures side track human dignity and agency. And without even realising it, people today in mainstream cultures collude with violence and prejudice.

As Dr Paul's Foreword expresses so well, there are many ways that these narratives of dominance need to be challenged. But unfortunately, his narrative also suggests that to engage in critique of the dominant politics we must also personally feel the weight of these systems and the actual damage they create. Only then do we proceed with the wisdom necessary to recreate new pathways.

Post-Colonial Contexts

Since the 1980s the early work of feminism, gay and lesbian studies, sociological analysis, liberation theology, creation spirituality, along with other cultural forms like wiccan and pagan philosophies have intentionally worked to deconstruct western systems of thought dominated by colonial forms of Christianity. Native studies have progressed on a parallel though independent path, seeking to articulate both Indigenous models as well as critiquing the colonial and western mindset.

At the community level people want to just get on with life. Having said this, the relationship between our leadership and education systems and the development of theory, models, and systems of thought are actually quite important. The model informs the training of native teachers and therapists, who work within the community, informing the next generation on ways forward. New ideas continue to evolve, and a feedback loop is created between higher studies, research projects, and the outcomes we need in community and family life.

At the base of community life, many issues come up that prevent people from getting on. Like Dr Paul says, prejudice creates barriers to access information, education, training, jobs, opportunities. Also, dogmatic attitudes towards issues like divorce and remarriage can create difficult situations for families who are suddenly restricted from participation in church or community.

Not that long ago in fact, living an Indigenous cultural wisdom across European nations and in the colonies led to inquisition and witch hunts. Indigenous values were conflated into the word 'pagan' by a largely corporate colonial and clerical Christianity. The term pagan originally meant 'of the country' and was used simply as a term to describe farming and regional communities. The term became more significant from the 13th century onward, when small city states were cropping up across European tribal nations that were being forged around fortress and self-defence structures. Ownership, control of land resources, defence, and an us vs. them value system became central to the development of corporate and civic law.

These trends remain central to contemporary law and the ways society is organized. The insidious nature of these forms of governance appear to pull everyone into the ways that life is defined. Remaining outside of this system is near impossible, such as might be felt by many native people who believe the Indian Act and First Nations identity provides a shelter from state based and international corporate systems. Unfortunately, native status is largely defined also in relationship to and by contrast with western corporate law and systems of government.

Yet we are seeing globally that there are push backs happening across many levels of community and corporate interests, including the ways that native people are using the corporate system to create legal and governance changes that are more in keeping with native values. While there is compromise involved by working within the present legal systems, there is also incremental progress being made towards self-governance if not self-government. These issues are central to the topic of this book. The reasons why may at first seem quite unfathomable. But in reality, Two Spirit issues and social political reality have always been deeply interrelated.

At one level, the status quo of colonial corporate culture including within Christianity was to control the masses through fear and intimidation. Lack of access to information was central to this strategy. Educational systems were restricted access as well, to provide only certain members of society with means to progress. By using identity categories to further restrict people's freedom of movement, access, and behaviour the ruling classes had another mechanism to control others. Although broad based restrictions usually backfire, because they restrict those in authority as well, the systems that develop tend to deal with these contingencies by increasing the privilege of the few.

Colonial culture and law made other categories that completely marginalized and quarantined native peoples while at the same time deployed prejudicial rules around various identities including ageism, gender conformity, and sexual ethics. Interwoven then are systems of thought and being, law and conduct, governance and identity. At the heart of the Two Spirit experience are always both social norms and personal experience.

Culture & Spirituality

In this way, Two Spirit defines the central issues for native rights – all of which rely on not only embracing social change but also personal freedom. During the 1990s we used to often hear the phrase 'the personal is political.' In many ways this is true, but not because the personal is contentious. Rather, the real issues are that western social political life and culture has become unhinged from humanity's heart which must rest within personal freedoms of conscience and self-defined identity.

This was also true in Mi'kma'ki, and applies to Two Spirit emancipation, and we can see how published Indigenous analysis has not yet caught up to articulating the extent of this trauma and recovery. In a way this book provides a window into this reflection on our histories and how we are digging our way out of the hole that colonisation created.

Today having a gay or lesbian child may create an awakening to parents, who suddenly realise that their community or church stance on 'homosexual issues' causes a great deal of harm. Parents and Friends of Lesbians and Gays (PFLAG) is one amazing group of people who exist to help parents in this transition towards acceptance and advocacy. Native social workers have most often stepped into this space to help families sort issues.

At the same time, while social conflict and small progress is being made, larger social movements are having a ground swell. In many ways change waits for the masses to shift, to move beyond past attitudes. Not only have Indigenous and First Nation spiritual ways had a resurgence this past two decades. Many other cultural forms that predated Christianity are arising once again in movements that seek to honour human and natural ecologies.

Many European Indigenous traditions are on the rise and are slowly being acknowledged within the colonial nation states of the Commonwealth. A great deal of reclamation is happening globally in a post-Christian, post-modern, and post-colonial environment. In many respects these movements sit outside of Christianity. But in other respects, there are forms of Christianity emerging that counter the colonial and western cultural bias that has dominated Catholic and Protestant approaches to faith and culture. In this sense, many today acknowledge that Christianity needs to unhinge itself from the dictates of western imperialism and colonial cultural bias.

Certain common values and approaches define Indigenous spiritualities. At the colonial level, native spirituality is discredited and subject to censure. But in postcolonial terms, native spirituality might be considered in a positive and generative sense. This occurs when we appreciate a reclaiming value such as with words like gay, queer, and aboriginal. It may seem obvious to us now, but in reality Mi'kmaq spiritual ways are integral to identity, and native spirituality is worthy of respect. This has not often, and not always been the case.

Words that were once used to marginalise and oppress people can sometimes become words of liberation. In this light, 'Indigenous' is a word that provides a degree of solidarity with other cultural and spiritual paths. Yet, as against corporate religions that 'do things by the book,' so to speak, Indigenous values highlight the ecological, personal, communal, regional, familial, and traditional. Indigenous values also appear to rely on the primacy of conscience and self-definition. There appears emphasis on communal and elder respect, and values of humility, listening, honour, and fairness or justice.

Among the western pre-Christian and contemporary spiritual paths that we have studied over the years we see many similarities among the older European cultural traditions and other Indigenous cultural forms of spirituality. Likewise, cross-cultural dialogue shows there may be similar elements within rituals, ceremonies, and teachings that are found within Mi'kmaq and other Indigenous paths. For instance, the Sacred Circle is common to many of these traditions and has universal dimensions within cultures around the world. Christians adopted the sacred circle, altar, and paschal fire and water in how churches were built upon four cardinal directions with the altar at the centre with baptismal candle and blessed water nearby. In Mi'kmaq, the Sacred Fire, Altar, and Water are at the heart of the Sweat Lodge Ceremony. An altar sits next to a Sacred Fire where the Elder Lodge Stones are heated and prepared. Water from a nearby river may assist during the Sweat.

Other cultural paths share similar symbols, such that, quickly enough, we learn how people have much more in common than we were led to believe. Again, quite intentionally prejudice generates intolerance that works to separate people from each other. Why? Because when we are separated and isolated, we become less powerful. Across these points of reflections we always ask, who benefits the most from keeping us isolated and ignorant of our strengths, capacities, and solidarity?

In certain respects, people's coming to terms with how their spirituality relates to others in a global world gives people a sense of common purpose across diverse traditions. Especially true when dealing with universal human problems like water rights and the survival of species including our own. Native spiritual paths have taken on a huge leadership role in stepping up to these global challenges. At the heart, yet again, are corporate interests that produce destructive circumstances.

While having invested many years into the formal study of Christian paths, out of respect and perhaps having grown a great deal, this book does not focus on these issues per se. Rather, our era appears focused on creating new pathways that honour traditional frameworks to make sense of the world we live in. As a Mi'kmaw person this means working in traditional knowledge systems to address current issues.

By traditional we mean that knowledge is alive, vital, and useful. Our models need to be pragmatic and effective, strategic and relevant. Traditional knowledge systems are integral, wholistic, connective, oriented to solution focused outcomes, and very robust. By robust we mean that traditional models are based in complex systems-values that observe ecologies, energies, and interactions over many generations. Our Elders carry this knowledge.

Indigenous science flows from traditional knowledge and is in many respects far advanced of most mainstream sciences. Western science is catching up as new generations challenge outdated bias and prejudice going back to the dark ages. Mi'kmaw science applies scientific method in a wholistic cultural landscape without the hang ups of western colonial histories.

Culturally speaking, our pre-colonial history demonstrates the implied use of complex systems theory within biological feedback models, including using principles of quantum physics inherent in our cosmology. This cluster of Indigenous values makes for a flexible ecological epistemology that is generative to scientific advancement. Clearly there are many points of convergence between science and Indigenous ways of knowing. Yet parallel to these insights, this book focuses on Two Spirit as an emerging social field of practice and discussion to provide a useful space to vision-quest the future. While we would like to remain in the positive here, there are also many conflicts that arise and that provide the context for advancement or regression.

Post-Colonial Spirituality

For many, the path toward mutual respect and integral spirituality is fraught with dangers. Over the past decade cultures have become that much more radical, unbalanced, and militant. White supremacy may also be part of this phenomena. Social media may provide platforms for organising militancy that did not have means before. At the same time, other social groups have grown toward self-acceptance and autonomy. Native cultures are no exception to this trend. There is much positive growth in minority cultures as well.

In times of upheaval we can see how spiritual authority in our culture ceases to exist within what we might call the colonial worldview. To understand post-colonial, we need to decolonise the body. Over the centuries in European nations, the colonial body was adrift and demonised by their own shadow issues that led to racial and natural genocide, ecological ruin, and now global climate degradation that threatens the narrow band of environmental conditions that actually sustain human life on earth. As we are seeing, our Elders have carried this Medicine all these many years from first contact until today.

The European cultures had generally placed personal authority into external systems of thinking, whether into Kings, Queens, Priests, Bishops or Pope. All led to the self-same outcome of disconnection and oppression. We can read this history in Elder Dr Daniel Paul's book, 'We Were Not the Savages.' And the story is clearly evident across a wider reading of history.

This same issue of diminishing personal authority is tied to global ecological genocide of the planet today. This underlying conflict of values exists across civil and corporate law. Modern forms of law are the children of canon law in the church that was written from Roman imperial law. The antithesis of gospel-based values, corporate law encourages disconnection and oppression. Land and water survival are at the heart of this story. And so is the Two Spirit Puoinaq.

Colonial teachings demand submission to external God-given authority in ministers or priests and bishops. Native teachings point to internal personal authority in humility and awakening, leading to integrity of thinking, speech, and action. Post-colonial models of spirituality nurture personal autonomy in ways that create harmony with nature.

Western nations are in identity crisis. Native nations are also caught in this same bind. We need to promote new models of spirituality based in integral studies. The epistemology of colonial verses integral ways of life is contrary in many ways. You either tend to side with one or the other, which influences your style and approach to both. To walk both ways in one path means compromise of both. You cannot walk in colonial and native spirituality at the same time without a great deal of compromise leading to hurt and suffering. The contradictions may cause profound trauma and suffering both psychological and social.

The only way that I have found to walk well is by shifting into a post-colonial spirituality that allows creative license and freedom to relate to various traditions from within a native cosmology. This allows for creativity, for honouring other paths and teachings, and for taking a more metaphorical and symbolic approach.

In similar ways, addressing the cluster of identity issues from gender to sexuality to race and Aboriginality requires a personal freedom of conscience. This can only grow and be nurtured in a society that is openminded. For this to happen, issues like prejudice, bias, violence, and stereotypes of personhood need to be resolved.

Scholarly analysis of the colonial histories across North America, Australia, New Zealand, and other nations shows the central issues of authority come about when personal identity confronts an unyielding corporate identity. Authority, agency, and autonomy are in this sense basic and essential human qualities that actually constitute the bedrock of international standards for human rights, including the united nations recognition of the rights of Indigenous peoples and nations, including the right to self-government.

Yet certainly these self-same rights are part and parcel of the Two Spirit path, as finding your way is certainly up to you, and at the same time living this way is inherently supported by a now robust human rights framework. But this understanding often appears invisible in local communities and workplaces. It is only by trial and error that we come to terms with harsh reality verses ideal rights and then we begin to write our own terms. The society around us begins to change, and in some ways, we move on to new awareness. But like my experience and the lives of many others who inspire this work, this takes time, patience, and a longsuffering commitment to family.

In this process of empowerment no one else can do this work for you. You can rely on family, tribe, and nation for support because we see these places as our origins and our future. Even when your family does not realise or have not awakened to supporting you as a Two Spirit, you can see past this moment towards a future of hope. This is your inherent, and your integral spiritual nature. You can see into the future in hope, in spite of all you see today. This capacity is part and parcel of Two Spirit Medicine and is central to the gifts that Creator provides to all children of earth.

Of Books & Medicine Bundles

This book is unique at this time in history. There is nothing quite like this in the literature on Two Spirit ways that combines the fields of Counselling, Psychology, Sociology, Sexology, Human Ecology, Spirituality, Cultural, and Indigenous Studies.

Most everything written about Two Spirit these days comes from an external perspective and rests only on an academic or professional purpose. We have not seen many works from practitioners of Two Spirit cultural ways. What is particularly unique about this book is that its intention is not only for academic, professional, or social service reasons per se. Yes, these are part of the picture, as we want this book to be as useful as possible. But in all truth this book is first intended as a culturally respectful help and guide to learn about Two Spirit Medicine ways from a Mi'kmaw perspective.

Written first for my nation's Mi'kmaw youth, and then for others who seek a deeper appreciation for Mi'kmaq Two Spirit ways, and then for others seeking to understand Two Spirit generally, and finally for those looking more broadly for insights into human sexuality and gender variance, spirituality and culture – this book is styled like a traditional Medicine Bundle. But like all bundles, it takes time to get to know the landscape. There are many layers to this mystery we call life. Youth and newcomers to these fields of knowledge will find this book challenging to read because we bring together many sources of insight and experience and we apply them to Two Spirit, Mi'kmaw, and First Nation issues.

Beware, this is not light reading and every page of this book raises difficult questions. On the other hand, get ready for some intimate and deep-thinking exploration of your personal, family, and cultural values. How exciting to engage at this level of personal and social medicine practice.

This is not easy reading, as the focus on your learning is always present. The purpose of this book is to inspire, challenge, and encourage exploration. We hope to help you open up new pathways to growth in both intellectual rigor as well as spiritual depth. This is asking a lot of you. We hope you are ready for this initiation into the Indigenous arts and sciences and Two Spirit ways. You must be on the threshold in some way or other, as otherwise you would not be reading this right now.

By drawing together scholarship, community identity, and practical insights this book is a Medicine Bundle with a punch. Every traditional medicine bundle can seem disorganised and symbolic, looking from outside. But once you learn more, every traditional bundle also has vision, logic, form, and content that makes sense and all fits together elegantly. Not to say this book bundle is elegant in its results, far from it, even though we have made our best effort to present a finished product for press.

In all truths, this book was allowed to emerge over two decades, perhaps longer in germination, and certainly focused over a twelve year period. This book is written by using a combination of professional, scholarly, personal, and poetic voice. The result is a collection of essays that are interwoven into an Ash tree basket, smudged by the sacred fires of Sage, Juniper, Tobacco, and Sweet Grass.

Elegance in form and function is a characteristic of ecological systems in nature. Human beings are the ones to mess this up extremely well. The oldest Medicine Bundles are passed down generationally. When receiving a bundle in this way, you are asked to sit for a long time, sometimes a decade or more. You are asked to listen and learn from the bundle as it is given. Over time the bundle and you become one being. But this takes time. This has been my experience and is reflected in this book in many ways.

This book is a kind of Medicine Bundle that works to undo some of the mess given by colonial inheritance and cultural crisis. By sitting a long time with this Bundle, we see how the inherent and integral logic of nature actually sets up the elegance of form and function once again. In spite of our mistakes and miss-wishes. We only need to listen, wait, and sit with the Medicines. But many people, especially youth, fail to realise how important is this sitting and listening.

You will find here in this Sacred Book-Bundle not only the problems. You will also find the solutions. If you take the models offered here, you will have a pathwork toward healing, recovery, and cultural revival already well underway. This book reflects this good work already happening among us. This is a therapeutic traditional Medicine Bundle of modern Puoinaq wisdom that comes from hard work, sacrifice, and heaps of inspiration; quite beyond in origins, as if coming from across the Six Worlds of our traditional cosmology and thus across eons of time.

When doing the final proof of this book it occurred to me that learning is a spiral. We begin in early life, learn some basic things. Then we keep learning the same lessons over and over again. Over the years we think we get all grown up. We might even think we know a lot of things! But in reality, we are simply doing the same circle since childhood. It came to me then that the images of our people already convey this wisdom. Like Elder Paul said, this book does not give new information per se, but finds a new way to combine teachings to speak to present day issues. This impression of the Bedford Basin stone carving suggests the spiral learning of life and the districts of the Mi'kmaq Nation. There are likely many meanings we can gather from this Sacred image.

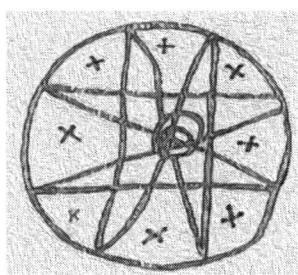

In keeping with the maritime ecology of Mi'kma'ki we developed an image below to convey the spiral learning found in this book. The journey begins with language, culture, ethics, and identity. The next layer explores spirituality, gender, sexuality, and ways of knowing. From these primary early learnings, we move to cultural reawakening, cultural teachings, oral tradition, and Elder's wisdom. From these sacred gifts, we explore ecology, ceremony as life, medicine teachings, and sacred sexuality. Continuing the spiral journey of life that began with language, culture, ethics, and identity we journey into deep memory, commitment, stories as healing and waking up. The last spiral of this book includes stories of our origins and living the Puoinaq Two Spirit Medicine path in living in service to family, humanity, and Mother Earth. All up this book includes four overlapping themes that spiral around six different cycles, with a total of twenty-four places along the circle or spiral. The basic four-point cardinal circle is the simplicity of self, our body. This is deeply informed by the natural symmetry of ecology.

We observe this sacred mystery of life within complex planetary bodies, solar orbits, humble sea shells, and in each other. We can see how a Sea Shell Spiral of Learning is in keeping with Mi'kmaw teachings and cultural ways. When reading this book, we suggest you consider how these themes evolve and grow in your awareness. Each subheading in the chapters does not mean that topics are covered under the heading. The headings introduce ideas in a creative flow to encourage reflection. Layered learning works within creative spirals. Revisiting your personal Sea Shell Spiral may help you to get a feeling for where you are in your journey of understanding. As we say elsewhere, take what you feel is good and useful for you. Disregard all the rest. There is a lot of wisdom here.

- Dr Joseph Randolph Bowers, 28 January 2019, M'sit No'kama Ta'ho.

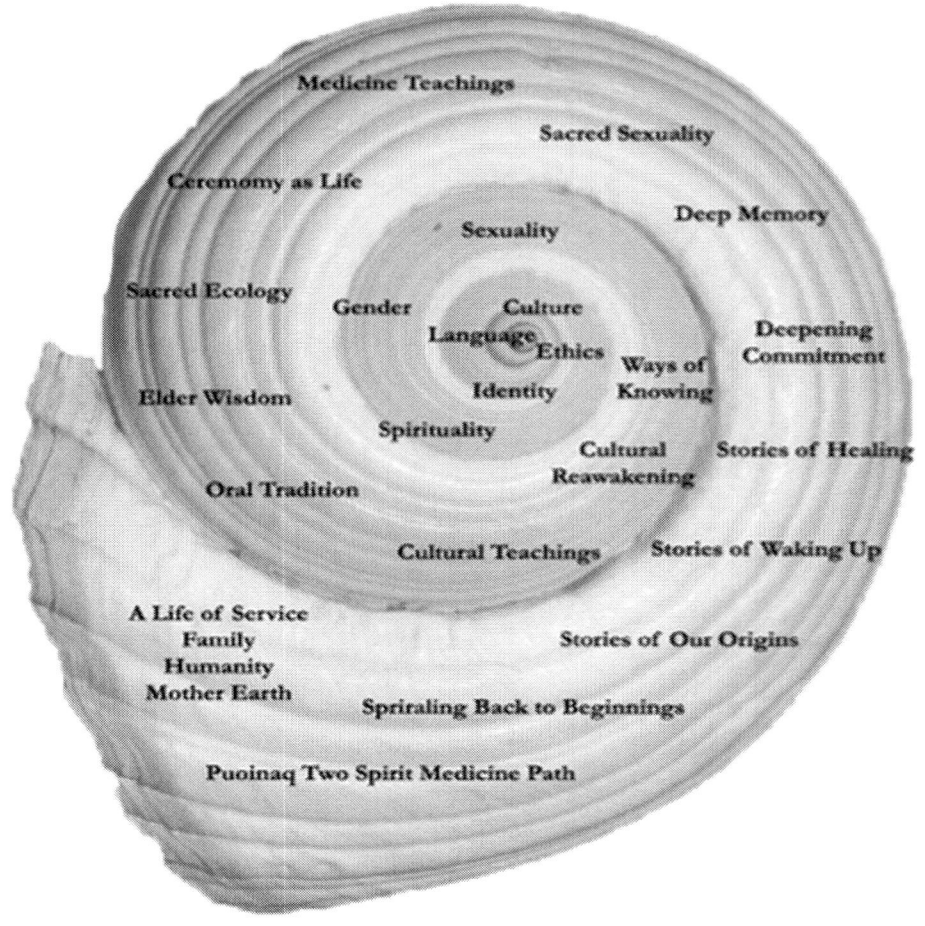

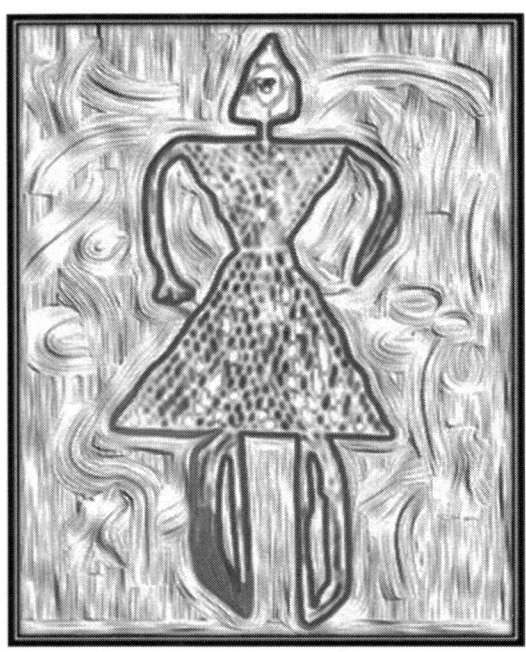

'We are the People of the Dawn, the Wabanaki. Our spiritual purpose is to Guard the Entry to the Sacred Circle, which sits in the East. In this way, we have tended the garden of Turtle Island... since the beginning of time...'

Mi'kmaw Tli'suti – Mi'kmaq Language

This section is written with a great deal of humility and ongoing reflection over the years. This process will continue. Please accept these notes as time-specific and unfinished. They reflect my own limited perspectives and search for meaning among the fragments of language received and the cultures of sharing language experienced.

The Mi'kmaq language is a dynamic and changing landscape of learning, growing, and creativity. The use of language in this book reflects this flexibility and appreciation for different dialects and individual forms and is decidedly non-dogmatic.

We ask your patience and forgiveness, if necessary, particularly during our era of language recovery and revival. We live in fascinating times when knowledge can be shared, and pan-Indigenous notions can be transmitted across vast distances. Living in Australia and learning language is certainly case in point. Dynamics of international marriages and relations of trade and commerce are part and parcel of our deep history also. Our native language reflects this.

The Mi'kmaq language grows from the roots of Algonquian linguistics and is kin with Cree, Deleware, and Ojibway (MRC 2017). Our nation sustains an oral tradition that was first recorded on stone and birch bark fragments in the form of pictorial representations. Hieroglyph and petroglyph writing developed out of the same spirit of creativity. The former grew particularly during early colonial encounter with Franciscan missions leading to prayers and scriptural texts translated into pictographs (Whitehead 1988).

During the 1970s the Francis Smith orthography added a new layer of clarity. Based on a phonemic principle and rooted in the early dictionaries of the 1800s the system is used widely today. But not consistently nor universally. Different dialects have existed throughout history, also true today even with the advent of distance communications. Certainly, language thrives where both consistency and diversity intersect and generate new forms of thinking and expression.

Two Spirit studies inspires the need to gather the Medicine Bundle of language. This is a brief and incomplete first impression gathered over ten years. We leave a comprehensive study to the younger generation of Two Spirit scholars and practitioners with more knowledge of these things.

Linguistically speaking, digging our-selves out of the Euro-centric flatland materialistic reductive gendered and racist worldview demands first appreciating Mi'kmaw wholistic cosmology as the basis of language and human relations. Notice we do not first say the need for understanding Mi'kmaw gendered relations. In fact, the vast majority of words and phrases in Mi'kmaq are non-gendered implying both/and rather than either/or. To prove this for yourself read a dictionary. A general verb-based emphasis on action is applied to any or all genders. This itself is fascinating because English places great emphasis on the noun.

Rather, in Mi'kmaq, people are described in pragmatic ways. For example, 'he chases men' is one of my favourites. Manly men and womanly woman appear descriptively in the language around what they do and what funny situations they find themselves in. Verbs are often tied to everyday tasks and roles. Men with women, women with men, men with men, and women with women may or may not be written about or described as *who they are* because the emphasis is on *what people do in acts of kindness or mistake*. You may not find someone described at all in colonial or culturally exposed settings, and if so, very briefly. Humility and propriety govern much of Mi'kmaw relations within and outside culture.

If during the colonial encounter gender tended to be 'hidden' among the Mi'kmaq (though gender as such cannot be viewed as a native concept per se, which technically is true when we study the colonial definitions of gendered roles in European cultures), how much more would a Mi'kmaq non-gendered, dual-gendered, or trans-gendered Two Spirit identity be hidden or remain simply not articulated? Indeed, many aspects of life are not raised or written because they simply do not become important in the culture until the colonial cultural clash demands self-examination, response, or resistance.

Puoinaq as Space for Vision

There is a poetry of being in the Puoinaq tradition. This is often referred to as shape-shifting. But part of this reality is the multi-dimension or many-meanings of being Two Spirit. This flexible description can apparently abide in any or all of the above dimensions of gender and relationship. One does not need be gay or lesbian in terms of sexual behaviour to be Two Spirit or a Puoinaq or both. This description can seemingly shape shift as well, i.e. move from being with male or female, appearing as male or female, and/or taking on the spirit-energy of totemic creatures, and/or taking on the more esoteric layers and personas of a Medicine Keeper, Pipe Carrier, Healer, or Seer.

While these insights arise from cultural learning, listening to elders, sitting with kin, and exploring sociological, psychological, and ethnographic reflections these insights also come from sitting with the Medicine bundle of language fragments.

Having not grown up with language, each word can take years of exploring, asking questions, listening to stories, and reflecting on meanings. Several reserve-based kin have told me that for this very reason we who have lived off reservation sometimes treasure cultural knowledge even more. While highly respectful to say of my desire to preserve and pass on knowledge, I would not come to the same conclusion as on reserve and off reserve are so unique for each person. Many regardless our background end up carrying these sacred medicines with great care and devotion.

Sitting with reserve-based grandmothers and fathers, cousins, aunts, and uncles, brothers and sisters, allows sharing stories and medicines. Anyone who studies Mi'kmaw language forms and culture will agree. This journey is incredibly rich from all sides given the depth and creativity of native associations, meanings, cosmology, science, poetry, and story.

Culturally speaking, in language we begin with Niskam, Great Spirit, who creates the cosmos and nurtures among the Old Ones of the People mediators and teachers in community that carry Sacred Medicines of knowledge systems, values, connections, and methods or skills. The Puoinaq are said to carry enormous powers of precognition, intuition, insight, wisdom, dream-knowledge, animal-knowledge, and ecological environmental-knowledge. We are said to live in deep ecology, deep connection, within all of creation. We are able to communicate and travel between the Six Worlds comprising Earth, Sky, Water, Under Earth/Water, Above Sky, and Stars or Ancestral World or the Summer Lands. Puoinaq as a word with its own history may or may not be linked or tied to notions of Two Spirit, or of spiritual power and identity variance. This connection may be contemporary.

Like Elder Dr Paul suggests, the links are plausible when we consider the broad values and intentions of the language and culture. Also, there appears to be layers of story that associate identity variance with the Puoinaq. We may not go so far as to say gender variance, or sexual difference. In so far as these latter concepts are highly charged by Eurocentric histories and colonial cultural origins.

But suffice it to say, if we had to stretch so far, we may admit that variance in identity could potentially in any given Mi'kmaw context include a person whose Puoinaq ways expressed or overlooked gender variance and/or sexual difference. In other words, a focus on who a person is remains less important than what that person does for family, tribe, and nation. Puoinaq in this sense is a person of power for the people. The word is associated with the action of a range of talents, perhaps including keeping family histories and marriages, healing arts, teaching, medicine keeping, herbalism, mysticism, spirituality, vision, connection with spirits, etc... How we serve and how we belong are the key concepts.

Personal layers of identity are only relevant when they are relevant, which is hardly ever in the sense that they may indeed never be spoken or written per se. To say Tom is gay or Two Spirit is absurd in this worldview. Rather, you may say yah well Tom chases men and he keeps the medicines. Go to Tom for the herbs you need. Oh yeah, Tom lives with Fred. They been together many years.

These kinds of connections may always have been or may be a contemporary acknowledgement of a layer of culture that has always been. Sometimes a people find obvious what was never quite clearly spoken before. But makes complete sense. I do not know if this is the case here. Not being dogmatic about history and tradition, my focus is on what people believe now, today, and how this helps people become stronger in good human values of kindness.

But the truth is that we can clearly say that Puoinaq is a word that was marginalised during colonisation and under Christian influence and was during a certain timeframe became associated with sorcery and witchcraft. This knowledge came to me late in this study and was quite a shock and surprise. In my innocent explorations this connection to European witch hunts and prejudice toward the arts and sciences of healing never occurred to me. This more extreme side of religious and cultural politics had been so clearly part of our history. Once this was raised naturally things began to make more sense.

This helped to explain from a sociological sense why and how gender, sexuality, and spirituality were marginalised in Mi'kmaw culture. In the Eurocentric colonial gaze, the three dimensions of sex, gender, and spirit are fused into one system of homophobic heteronormative legalism. Thus, the contemporary uptake of Puoinaq is more than simply relevant but is potentially deeply healing.

Much the same dynamic happened in European tribal nations throughout the middle ages as the power of the church grew and imposed violence upon the keepers of medicine, lore, story, and cultural wisdom – women, elders, and gender variant gay and lesbian people whose place in societies around the world tends toward keeping sacred these creative cultural arts. And yes, the historical record shows clearly that gay men were persecuted along with witches, midwives, and anyone suspected of or feared to challenge the dominant male hetero-exclusive exercise of power. My PhD had me examine this history for a full year, leading to the first chapter of the thesis looking at how European cultures treated same-gender love since the medieval era to today.

Therefore, from analysis of western constructs to holding a culturally Indigenous scholarly view, Puoinaq as a word, concept, and cultural repository holds huge potential for exploring the healing of our nation. Ironically and humorously Mi'kmaw people might say 'Puoinaq'jij' to catch the irony of 'Little Person of Power,' or 'Person of Little Power' to push the loving joke a bit further. Or likewise to acknowledge youthfulness in these ways. To call oneself a Puoinaq'jij is quite appropriate, we are always students and learners on the path.

The word 'Puoinaq' is useful to suggest a wide range of meanings as well as the higher degrees of the Two Spirit phenomenon that embrace spirituality and medicine traditions. These are indeed 'great' because they are of great value to families, tribal groups, and the nation. What is great to the Mi'kmaq is what serves family, tribe, and nation in humility of purpose. You find this paradox of humility in every teaching.

As one Elder said, when the Two Spirit are given a place of honour and respect not only will they serve the nation with great humility, but the nation will also become strong again. Implied here is the relationship of the people to their Medicine Keepers, and to their sense of embodiment and freedom to love one another in relationships of deep abiding respect and honour. Also implied are how the symbolic place of the Puoinaq represents vital knowledge systems, ways of knowing, and practices of culture and learning that are part of nation building. While these ways of knowing were diminished and marginalised during colonisation elders suggest these ways were never lost. These ways are reawakening now. Coming back to the Elder's Circles along with the Sacred Pipes.

We cannot overlook how the notion of Two Spirit emancipation among the Elders also suggests the reality of how these same Elders were subject to the rape and violence of residential schools, and how children today are taken away in even greater numbers into off-reserve families, many of whom are not Indigenous. Disenfranchisement happens in a number of ways and perhaps Two Spirit people are seen as one of the more vulnerable groups among the people, targeted for generations during this central battle against European invasion and cultural genocide.

Language and Cultural Revival

Because the colonial-gaze, as monolithic as it was, viewed the Mi'kmaq people as having no religious beliefs and sought to convert us to Christianity, the power dynamics of survival sent cultural teachings underground and abroad. Wise and astute Grand Chief Membertou and 21 members of his family in a sign of good faith became baptised in 1610. Now there are layers of Catholicism in our history overall. St Anne became our patron saint being a grandmother. Her regard says more about our people than about the Christian tradition that does not tend to elevate Anne to such a degree.

Many today view the choice of Membertou as a benevolent gesture that was never meant to suggest conversion to Christianity per se, but as nurturing collegial political relations with the King of France and his governors. In the context of the day, the French-Mi'kmaq relationship was indeed collegial, as many families intermarried, and the rule of law was in certain ways bilateral for that brief time in history.

If the baptism of the Grand Chief was meant as gesture of good will or more, and whether he understood the implications is highly speculative. Given the complexity of symbolism and the difficulty in translating the meaning of Latin baptismal rites into Mi'kmaq which is a work that has never been completed to date, it is more than likely that Membertou was at a distinct disadvantage.

In the post-colonial sense at least, it is perhaps more important to acknowledge how Christian and Catholic baptism was viewed by the French, and then later subverted to other ends under British colonial rule, and then used by Catholic missionaries and the latter establishment of Catholic churches on all of the reservations across the territory. To a careful look into how contemporary Catholic and Christian relations with the Mi'kmaq are managed. This analysis and critique of colonial Christian-Mi'kmaq relations are quite another story indeed, and a story that dearly needs to be researched and written by future Mi'kmaw scholars.

Not exactly incidentally, some 42 years later my French ancestor Michel Richard arrived in 1652 and began a long line of intermarriage among the Mi'kmaq of the Bear River and Acadian bands of the Mi'kmaq Nation. Our heritage is now 14 generations later and is documented with the Mi'kmaq Resource Centre. In Mi'kmaw symbolism, 7x2 generations is significant, a turning point. In a sense our current generations are pivotal in ways that may not be obvious to many living in our era. Suffice it to say we are like all generations the 7th generation that is spoken of in prophecy and story.

The prophecy suggests that when the medicines come home to the people, a great time of healing and nation building will begin. But here again, the same can be said for every generation and we are all of the 7th generation! However, for me personally this skin-time and the fact of the history has made me stop and consider, what ways can I make a difference in this life? Why am I here? What can I do for my people? Perhaps all youth need to ask these questions. These questions really do open up vision quest and truth be told the important part is not finding your answer. The more important aspect is living your questions.

The ancient practices of Mawio'mi or gathering during the summer abundance at Chapel Island and Merigomish continue from ancient times where the Chiefs of the nation gather to discuss national issues and govern tribal boundaries and sustainability issues for fishing and hunting. Colonisation has changed some things, but not everything.

Language is Culture, Ecology, Spirit

The Puoinaq have various roles according his/her capacities and skills. For instance, combined with these traditions is L'nui-nsisun – Herbal Medicine of the People, given pride of place among the Medicine Keepers, this is first a practical art for health and wellness.

Secondly for emotional and social wellbeing. Always for spiritual insight. For example, Welin'qewe'l Msiku – Sweet Grass has astringent purification aspects with great ceremonial value, particularly in honour of Ancestors and thanksgiving or gratitude. Also helpful with depression, especially during winter months. Many other herbs hold valuable properties being recorded these days and celebrated more so among the people.

Traditional ways of life were and are governed by practicality and personal skill, strength or ability. What one is drawn to do for the family or group is often encouraged. Better to have a happy camper than someone grumbling and annoying. Things are often taken as the path of least resistance in allowing diversity of behaviours in fun, laughter, and good relations.

Respect is the primary value across every relationship, between people or with animals and nature. While not actually nomadic the Mi'kmaq had distinct tribal territories that were divided by the Chiefs and ratified for the sake of sustainability in fishing and hunting. For instance, my family is said to have gathered on the coast during summers in numbers up to 300 or so people. The abundance and climate allowed for good fish and game, foraging and sustainable practices.

To be nomadic suggests no organisation or territorial values. Imagine 300 people dispersing for the winter months, tracking to their traditional winter grounds only to find another family camped. I'm sure that must have happened now and then. But the results of such mistakes could be catastrophic. To survive the winter with reduced game and fishing in extremely harsh permafrost conditions would place extra burdens on the ecology, likely leading to starvation of members of a family group.

To prevent this eventuality as well as the risk of injury from argument and conflict among people the elected Chiefs and Elders would gather first thing after proper greetings and hold Council for the summer dealing with important business. Whose winter grounds were good this year, who needs a new location, what was the game doing and how were our kin of the Bear Nation or Wolf Nation? The predators and game would be discussed, the issues of the land and regeneration of the bush was considered. Plans were made, and agreements struck on who would go where for the winter months ahead. Hardly nomadic. This was an advanced form of consensus civic organisation and sustainable governance based on a scientific model of human and environmental ecology.

My family for example has connections between the coast of the South Shore and Bay of Fundy of Nova Scotia. Our winter grounds were back near Wildcat reservation, around what is now Queens County. In the 1650s Michel Richard settled his family at Belle Isle near Port Royal. Over time the family embraced Mi'kmaw ways and remained loyal during the worse parts of the Acadian Expulsion.

While much was lost, much remains. Men's roles today might look a bit different but still celebrate similar energies and skills. These traditionally include hunting, making bows, arrows, lances, axes, tools, cradle boards for infants, and stone pipes. Men learn the arts of making shields, spears, fish-traps, canoes, snowshoes, cooking implements, and knives. From today's view, I don't think fixing cars, machinery, computers, carpentry, chopping wood, or driving trucks and snow ploughing are all that different jobs for men. Men today share many roles with women like they always have.

Not always exclusive to gender women's focus includes setting camp, carrying whatever was kept between camps, preparing hides, skinning animals, food preparation, food preservation, weaving baskets, making woven mats, rushes, Birch bark dishes, and containers, making clothing, cording snowshoes, keeping fire, gathering wood, and during harvest and foraging the gathering and preservation of food stuffs.

Women took care of infants and children and all together took responsibilities for raising children as a village among an extended family kinship system. Today women will keep the home going in similar ways. Modern demands on family life hold different but similar challenges. When you consider how robust our Ancestors were to live in Wigwams and cook on the open fire every day, we have much to be thankful for, and much to learn.

One fascinating story that I remember is how a certain woman felt sorry for her partner who she saw had great difficulty going from trap to trap and carrying game back to camp. He had to cross this river to get to the other side of the lake, then back again, meanwhile a trap went off in a distant location. He had to walk far and expend valuable time and energy. This is what people did for generations. She pondered this problem a long time and funny enough she had three dreams, one dream each night, over a period of time. She dreamed how to make a canoe. Each dream gave her more ideas and clarity. When she woke from the third dream, she knew she had to build this container from Birch bark because in her dream she had seen her partner travel the lake and collect game that was put in the centre of the canoe, easily carried back to shore and brought to camp.

She got her partner to help build the canoe, much to his dismay. The story goes into great detail in each step of the process, sad we cannot share that here. Then when the canoe was ready, she told him what to do, she had to tell him everything of what to do.

He gingerly got one foot into the canoe and it rocked side to side. He jumped out in fear! She told him to get back in, that he had to get in this way, and how to sit, and what direction to face. He listened and eventually after much to do, she got in the canoe and paddled him across the edge of the lake first staying close to shore because he was still so fearful.

She knew it would work OK. Her dream told her so, and she knew how to make a very good Birch container for cooking, keeping fresh food, and setting delicate fern greens in a smaller Birch bowl inside a larger pot of water to steam them just right. Her dream was true.

The story continues through their adventures in that first ever canoe, and to the place where she settled many leagues up river to a lake she had never seen before, to the special island where loons raised their young. She decided to rest and to die on that island, which she did, and she was happy. I read a similar story to this in Whitehead (2002) and surprising how the stories overlap in detail. This is often the case with our oral traditional stories. Language is like this, as words have meanings that carry across distance and time. It is a spiritual gift, language.

Two Spirit realities arise from the mists of time through this same spiritual ecology of story and language, this culture of language. This is family life. Today's world might challenge this central value, but the Two Spirit role upholds this value in service to the family. This is our primary role and purpose. This is the underlying meaning of the language and spirituality of our Two Spirit cultural ways.

The words below or phrases were collected over a 10-year period. Many do not use the Francis Smith orthography. They appear as they were given, and this seems more respectful at this time. Also, I am not qualified to change them into a certain orthography.

As language is personal and meaningful, and as a Mi'kmaw Two Spirit doing my best with the little resources available, please accept this sharing of language with my respect and deepest humility.

We leave the tasks of linguistic organisation and sorting 'right from wrong' forms to the young ones who are interested in that sort of thing. John Sylliboy (2017) does the nation a great service in his thesis that honours traditional Mi'kmaw ways and arising from his first language speaker's knowledge. His work is instructive and inspiring. We have the pleasure of reading his thesis as we finish this book, and while he expresses things in a different manner the underlying treatment of language and culture appear fairly similar and parallel. This gives me a sense of humility and respect for the actual robust nature of Mi'kmaw languages, cultures, and spiritualities that can bridge the distances between first language speakers and those of us who grew up off reservation and without this wealth of language. It is extremely telling what the author says about the emergent nature of knowledge. 'Conceptualizing two-spirit within Mi'kmaw language and storytelling to understand it within a cultural worldview, is part of the transformation within the flux, a source of developing new knowledge as part of a cultural continuity (2017, p. 84).

Beginning the path many years ago not knowing one word that referred to Two Spirit, the most immediate impression is wow. Incredible. And here is a book to reflect our identity and build strong families… This is so amazing.

The following word list is fairly broad, and this is intentional, in the sense that Mi'kmaq is a contextual verb-based and fluid language that relies on an extremely rich wholistic, cognitive, ontopoetic, and open-hearted consciousness. This list is hardly definitive and is itself an expression of continual reflection and learning. Sitting with one word can last many years, even decades. New associations and meanings, the addition of prefixes or suffixes can blow apart limited perspectives and open up whole new vistas.

This reminds me of sitting with a Mi'kmaw man at Eskasoni who shared with me how one of my given names in language, Paq'tism, is reflecting the actual sound of a wolf tearing into the flesh of an animal. His description and how he said the word shocked and excited me, giving me a whole new appreciation for the descriptive, alive, dynamic, graphic, symbolic, and musical nature of Mi'kmaq.

In English this quality is called onomatopoeia, i.e. 'the imitation of sound.' But fascinating to realise that the word's actual roots come from Greek where it means 'making or creating names.'

The cultural role of Shieldwolf and from 'Randolph' in its ancient Indigenous Teutonic linkages suggests the wolf who serves the Alpha by scouting ahead and returning to the pack, letting them know when safety or danger lies ahead. In Mi'kmaq the Paq'tism has an Alpha quality but can be associated with other roles and is a word for wolf generally. The scout in Mi'kmaq are navigators across land, sea, and by mapping the stars. Orienteering is a key survival skill that all Mi'kmaq once learned. The scout sought good hunting grounds, looked for dangers, read the signs of animal migration, and sensed the seasonal changes leading to change of camp. Like John Sylliboy (2017) suggests of his role as an educator, we have also taken these roles of seeking far and wide for wisdom as a healer, counsellor, and therapist drawing potentials for change among those we work with and for our people.

In Mi'kmaq we see and feel intuitively an incredibly creative emergence of meaning, sound and story; imagery and imagination; moving pictures and narrative developments; twists and turns and deep ecological associations that ebb and flow like the Fundy tides. It is important to realise that these insights come from a non-first-language speaker, as we feel that if we can grasp these layers of complexity and can respect deeply the Mi'kmaw worldview simply from the rare fragments we are given, then surely anyone can learn and be enriched. Mi'kmaw language has a vital part to play in knowledge generation in Canada and around the world. Mi'kmaw language has a cross-cultural and global significance that in fact contributes to many emerging fields of science and practice let alone having a key role to play in the present global need for robust linguistic and scientific frameworks that can ensure ecological sustainability and environmental regeneration.

Regarding sources for words began during the early 1990s. In a sense, my life long scouting for reconnection as a displaced Mi'kmaw person led to collecting language fragments over many years. The first that I remember finding was a word that was described as 'he chases men.' I cannot say how that one word opened up validation and relief in heart and mind. As simple and strange, and funny as it sounds this is true. My hope is that this word list will help Mi'kmaw youth in future and will inspire more study and learning to build our families and inner resilience. Sources for most of these words are lost to time as they were often written on scraps of paper and transcribed into files over a twenty-eight-year period. Many were found online, others were given in discussion with friends and family, others gleaned from media and then social media when that emerged.

Many people appear to be searching for one word to say, 'Two Spirit' in the Mi'kmaq language. They hope to find something that proves the existence of a tradition from the past. We used to seek this, but over the years we have come to appreciate a cultural perspective. This point of view feels family and community contexts and a sense of timelessness that exists in the now with our Ancestors. Language may come to express Two Spirit more directly over time, and as we begin to heal from colonialism and move on into our own ways, but this is a journey perhaps even a bit of a vision quest for our generations living now. As such, the following word list provides context not specifics per se. Broad contours rather than detailed images. Whether we like this or not, it appears that the Elder's Sacred Council is still in discussion over these matters.

Mi'kmaw Words Associated with Identity, Gender, Sexuality, and Two Spirit

As stated throughout this chapter, this list is not exhaustive nor definitive. This is a work in progress that we hope will be further developed in future by others interested in linguistic studies. We have inserted a star (*) to indicate words more directly associated with observed usage for LGBTIQ2S+ meanings. Again, we note that observations of more direct word usage reinforce the acknowledgement of a non-gendered and non-sexualised cosmology within traditional culture among the Mi'kmaq people.

Espi-Saqmaw	Great Chief
E'pit	Woman, Female
*E'pite'suamuksit or Epitejijewe'k	He Has the Appearance of a Girl, Effeminate Boy (Sylliboy 2017)

E'pitewa'teqa	Woman's Fashion / Way of Appearing
Geenumu Gessalagee	Incorrect past translation of 'He Loves Men.' Literal correct translation is 'One Loves Men.' Identified only in published literature by non-native authors the phrase was incorrectly assumed to reflect internal cultural associations with gender and/or sexuality variance and/or with Two Spirit Mi'kmaq. Original publication was Roscoe (1998, p. 214). To date, Sylliboy (2017) provides the most detailed published analysis. Sylliboy aptly shows that the phrase is linguistically incorrect, incomplete, non-gender specific, and does not reflect historical nor contemporary language use within the culture of the Mi'kmaq.
Genum Genuumu Gesallagee	He Loves Men or literally Man Loves Men, or implied '(a) Man (who) Loves Men,' Here Genum is used for Man, to represent 'he'. Offered by Sylliboy (2017, p. 70) as a linguistic correction to Roscoe (1998). However, as Sylliboy suggests, 'There is no evidence of any validation for its use' within the culture. Sylliboy suggests other terms like Kistele'k have been demonstrated to be in common use.
Ila'lati	Heals, Repairs Someone i.e. physically, mentally, or spiritually
Jinisjam	Great Spirit
Ji'nm	Man, Male
Ji'nmuit	Is a Man
*Ji'nmue'sm	Man Chaser, Likes the Company of Men, Referring to women usually, used for both genders (Frank Meuse, early correspondence), may suggest humour and simple social observation with no perjoritive meaning observed
Ji'nmu'qamigsit	Acts Like a Man
Ji'nmutagn	Manhood

*Kepmitelsi (noun)	I Am Proud, I am Filled with Pride, adopted by youth of Eskasoni First Nation during 2016-17 Pride celebrations (Social media, and Sylliboy 2017, p. 103)
Kesalul	I Love You
Kesaluet	Loves, To Love
Kesatk	Likes, Loves, Is Fond Of
Kinap (singular), Kinapk (plural)	Gifted, Gifted (man/woman), Great Warrior, Hero, Of Higher Power, being born with powers or taking on or growing in powers through life
Ki'nupsom or Ginup Some	Two Spirit, transliteration
*Kisiku	Elder (old man), also Elder (old woman), also observed in use for person(s) identified by Elders as Two Spirit and in rare cases given as part of a traditional name
Kisiku'skw	Elder Woman (old woman), often felt to be redundant to add 'skw' where the meaning is known
Kisikui'skwewit	Is An Older Woman
Kiste'k	Beaten, Punished, Sex with Her, Banged her (slang)
*Kistele'k	Acting Oddly, to describe gay or lesbian, as a pejorative among youth, in colonial or homophobic context may include notion of deviance, sin, shame, or stigma (Sylliboy 2017)
Lnu, L'nuk (noun), L'nuwey (adjective)	Native, Aboriginal, First Nation Person
*L'pa'tujewe'k	Acting Like a Boy, also with girls as such in a tolerant usage without the derogatory sense
Migigneqwinu	Strong Person
Mimajuinu	Human Being, Person
*Mu'k epitejijewey	Don't Act Like a Little Girl (or sissy)
Negm	He/She, Him/Her

Negmow	They/Them
Nemijgami	Grandfather, term of respect and endearment for an older man
Nepiteket	Healer, Curer
Niskam or Gisu'lgw	Creator
Nitap	Friend
Ogoti	Dear, Friend, used for affectionate term between spouses
*Puoin (singular), Puoinaq (plural)	Being or Person, People with Power; Power to heal, cure, or lead; Power to pull apart, change, transform; Associated with shape changing, trickster, shifting between various human and/or totemic capacities; Contemporary use for Two Spirit among Mi'kmaq Two Spirit community including the Wabanaki Two Spirit Alliance
Skw	Woman, Female, Young Woman
Ta'pu Jigaqamij (singular), Ta'pu Miijaqamijjk (plural)	Literally words for Two and Spirit, not of common usage

Editor's Note: The quotes before each chapter throughout the book are taken from Bowers (2013) Sacred Teachings from the Medicine Lodge.

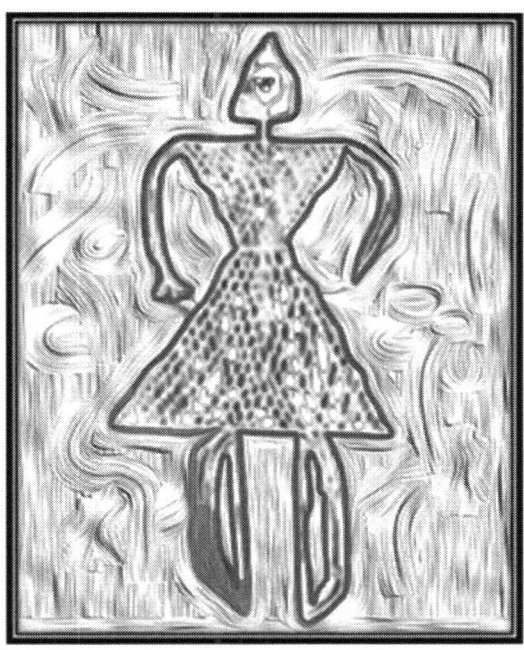

'We can become deeply connected with the plants, trees, and weather systems; the rocks, hills, valleys and natural features of the land and water bodies; and the winged, finned, four legged, flying and crawling creatures who live and share this Earth World.'

Two Spirit Ethics

Pjila'si, welcome, come in, sit down. Welcome to our sacred fire in this humble wigwam.

Committing these ideas to writing began with talks around the kitchen table at Whycobah First Nation during the summer of 2007. At the time, I was visiting the summer gatherings and accepted invitations to several native reservations across the region. The reason for my trip from Australia was to reconnect with heritage and culture, to learn from the elders, and to answer some long-standing questions that remained within me since my father passed over during 1997. The summer of 2007 was a pivotal time for me because many of the pieces came together. It is now 2017, we seem to go in decades by seven…

The year 2007 was important not the least of why was to confirm that elders today remain steadfast in supporting Two Spirit identity within native communities. Discussions with several elders led to understanding that Two Spirit is respected in many ways. The rest of this book explores these meanings and suffice it to say that visits and discussions invited a process of recording notes from learning and keeping teachings with care. Two Spirit Medicine traditions awakened over time. But writing a book was an entirely scary prospect.

Many have asked me what my intentions are. After examining my views, I am often told to continue on this path because 'your focus is pure in heart.' This message conveys the strength and honour of Mi'kmaq culture and family values. The statement also tells me to ponder the social politics involved in Two Spirit relations.

True for all native teachings primarily people want to know that you will respect native ethics, honour cultural wisdom, and respect safety for family and children. Ethics are central in Mi'kmaw culture, family, and for children, women, men, and elders. The best way to describe this is with boundaries. Putting things plainly, I believe strongly in personal and social boundaries that help keep children and vulnerable people safe from exploitation, abuse, and harm.

Relations of Respect

Boundaries of conduct and behaviour are essential to healthy lifestyles and to preventing issues of violation and trauma. Naturally, consenting adults can and will do whatever they please. However, when making these pivotal decisions about our intimate and sexual conduct we ought to consider that our behaviour will impact on many other people around us. In today's world where freedom is associated with absolute personal licence to do whatever you want, there can be dire consequences. Boundaries relate to not only close relations but to the nation and global human family. We might say that good boundaries promote and nurture our ecology, in unity with our planet.

Mother Earth is part of our intimate family relations. This is a basic traditional teaching - an insight from ancient times that speaks of our interdependence on life itself. We are not individuals bent on personal gain. We are members of a family and nation and required to act accordingly with respect and honour.

Entering into knowledge in whatever forms adds deeper responsibility to the mix. If anything, people can be more likely to side with caution and become more conservative in their values and processes of decision making. Wisdom is like this.

The more knowledge we have the longer it takes to make a decision - just ask a traditional elder to answer a question. If you hear back from them within six months you are quite surprised. Often, they may reflect on your question for a year or two. And this is partly because they will go away and think through everything they already know, and then they will do their research, ask questions of others, and form a basis for a deeper discernment. Going a full cycle of moons may give different perspectives on any question.

Boundaries are also about ethical and moral responsibilities. This is serious stuff. Readers might want to skip this part. But the truth is that these points are the key to this topic and this book. Two Spirit reality is not a joke, nor a big party. Though we love a nice party. At the core, Two Spirit is a sacred path of profoundly moral and spiritual teachings that govern right conduct and right action.

This is an important and valuable point. There are those who take the party path, and there are many gatherings where sex, drugs, and rock and roll play a larger part while sacred ceremonies may also happen. Nothing new really as Catholics or other cultures do the same thing. People are people. And life is also meant to be enjoyed. To have fun is good. Also, good to celebrate and uphold the sacred. Elders and Pipe Carriers may tend to avoid places and spaces unsafe for the sacred, unless they have a rather specific purpose in mind like education.

Naturally, Two Spirit realities for some people has little or nothing to do with the medicine path. This path may not exist in any given community, and knowledge comes and goes over time. There may be an unusual or rare quality to these teachings, though they are gaining strength as more people open up and take on these ways of being. Awakening is a path that is personal and social, familial and national, in dimensions.

For me, being a keeper of medicines in today's world naturally led to a solitary path that grew into being a practitioner and healer, teacher, and therapist. From solitude the path reunites with others. Solitary life guides and gives time to listen and builds strength and resilience.

Sitting with the medicines takes time in and of itself, just learning to live and commune with one herb can take several years of learning. Foraging and keeping a garden have taught me so much about culture and spirituality. These are only two practical examples.

Therefore, the teachings offered here about Puoinaq Two Spirit, and spirituality in general, may not directly be found in any given community. You may find these teachings implied. Something may feel familiar. That is because these teachings are like a mirror of clear water. When you look at the water you see the lake or pond. You see reflected your embodiment, and if you look more deeply, your spirit. You also see the sky or trees. Above the trees you may see the Eagle fly over. Above the Eagle you might notice the clouds and shape of the moon. Hidden in the reflection you may notice the feminine qualities of water, the strong masculine forms of cloud formations, the stately man-like trees, and the feminine softness of the moon. All this from looking at the surface of water. You find the pathway to seeing the Puoinaq through the reflections of the water.

These teachings may exist in special places. They are accessible when you look closely enough, and as you hold on to solid values. You can fall off the path by losing any one of these things, because these teachings only surface in nurturing consistent effort and sacrifice. Especially true today when we are swayed by so many different ideas and values. It is not that we need to become sheltered. Nor over protective. It is simply that nurturing solid native teachings around Two Spirit spirituality takes a great deal of effort, consistency, and sacrifice. But for those on the path, sacrifice is joyful and simply part of living in beauty. Boundaries are a good example.

Boundaries are about clarity in beliefs. For example, many thinks that Two Spirit is simply another native catch phrase for gay, lesbian, bisexual, transgender, or intersex. This is simply not true and not very helpful.

Two Spirit is a quite distinct identity and pathwork. This work on the path of family life stands apart from European labels. The historical names or labels of gay, lesbian, etc., speak mostly to sexual conduct. Gay means you have sex with men. Lesbian means you have sex with women. Bisexual that you have sex with either or/both. Transgender does not specify the object of affection. A trans person may be gay, lesbian, or heterosexual. Intersex means having the physical genitalia or aspects thereof from both genders in one body. Meanings may also develop around gay culture, lesbian culture, etc., so that the meanings are much broader than sexual disposition. But in common usage the sexual conduct of the person is the focus.

These terms may be helpful but there is also a sense that they are foreign to native cultures. Their emphasis is on the noun. They tend not to focus on ethics and relationships. They tend to be disconnected from the heart.

Reconnecting is actually helped by re-associating the person to the family, the self to culture. This is a native way of setting boundaries back into natural order. Boundaries are one of the most essential parts of sexual and intimate relationships between people. Nature governs her boundaries with great care and creativity.

Boundaries form a place of safety within which two people can explore their minds, hearts and bodies. Understanding 'my space' verses 'your space' is a basic human life-skill learned during the early years of infancy as the child comes to distinguish between parent and self, other and self. This innate relational boundary becomes important as children grow and explore 'my friend' and 'your friend' and within this the variations and complexities of human relationships.

Native and nature-based culture often sees and celebrates we-relations, our-family, our-nation. Not so much me, my, and I the focus of native culture is we, us, and ours. These perceptions come through during childhood development where self-identity is formed in secure attachment to relationships.

Healthy early relationships between youth and young adults that enter into sexual experimentation also tend to express a strong sense of privacy, personal space, sharing with someone special, and containment of the experience within normal social boundaries. As people grow older these boundaries around intimacy tend to remain strong and come to define the choices young adults and adults make through commitments to having children with a partner, marriage and/or long-term commitments to stay together, and similar arrangements. Two Spirit people undergo a similar human developmental path.

One difference between the developmental paths of Two Spirit people and others is that the Two Spirit person might have the capacity to form intimate relationships with people of either gender. Some are drawn to one or the other, or both. In native culture and during childhood this capacity to love both genders can form even deeper bonds of attachment that can at times be unusual and welcomed or a bit disconcerting to one of the parents or other adult carers in the child's world. Likewise, if there are issues, the innate capacity may lead to fracturing of relationships with adults who may not understand the nature of Two Spirit children and youth.

There is a sense that the Two Spirit person may represent a third gender, although we are happy to simply say that the Two Spirit person represents a different way or path in life. And by suggesting three genders we remain unhappy. We do not actually want to promote the mainstream binary – gender is not all there is in nature.

Nature is diverse and exists in circles. Even tall grass and reeds and tree stems and bark come in straight lines that are relatively easy to form into circles. The tops of trees like the hair on a native man's head arches back down to the earth forming a complete circle. Even straight men are circles.

Women embody the circle in so many ways, they are more familiar with this power. Their intuitive sense knows the Two Spirit way is sacred, because their embodiment exists closer to this form and being.

Women are the first Medicine. Men are the second Medicine. Women nurturing and becoming masculine in spirit are the third Medicine. Men nurturing and becoming feminine in spirit are the fourth Medicine. Women loving women may be a fifth, men loving men a sixth, and Two Spirit beings a seventh Medicine. The highest or more complete medicine way is combining and transcending the basic energies of existence within one being, a learning that seems to happen over many skin-times. In the utmost simplicity, loving kindness and the basic human capacity to love another being is truly at the heart of all sacred Medicine. The Seven Medicine Two Spirit Teaching is quite important to ponder. This teaching comes from the

Mi'kmaq Marriage Pipe. There is much wisdom here. All other variations exist in this teaching. Diversity in creation is affirmed.

Relational Norms

From strong boundaries based in beliefs and values our approach to sexual ethics generally holds monogamous relationships in high esteem. Whether gay or straight, bi-sexual or transgender, intersex or Two Spirit, in my observations of people over many years and in study of human sexual behaviour we are relatively convinced that the norm and the preference is for long-term one-on-one relationships.

In some cases, we have seen people maintain healthy and long term sexual familial relationships between more than two people, but these tend to be rarer and more exceptional. Simply put, to reach maturity and depth most people need to grow in intimacy over several years with one special person. This is where we get the notion of a soul mate. Add another person to the couple and things get fairly complicated.

As well, longevity and maturity cannot be easily attained through temporary encounters. Many people will argue this point and may have fooled themselves into believing they have attained nirvana. All I can say is each to her own. But we are not convinced, and these views are likely shared by the majority of human beings on the planet. For whatever reasons people form couple bonds, and this is one of the primary circles in nature.

Many say that marriage between a man and woman is normative. In terms of numbers this may be true. In relation to human diversity, people are people.

Marriage is another topic indeed. Mi'kmaw marriage tended to be more flexible and relied on adult consent, consent of family, and then also consent to end a relationship if/when needed. Binding legal codes did not exist to such a degree. Raising children and sharing of resources was more communal.

Couple relations breaking down would create awkward times but may not pull apart relationships in many cases. Today things are a bit different under

Christian rules and legal frameworks. These impact on native cultures. Ironically gay marriage provides an interesting variation on the theme, just enough so that people today may ask questions about how they can form and maintain a couple relationship. Once gender is not so opposite, male verses female, and once you mix things up a bit, gender becomes less important and just part of life. People are people, and most of us are mixed up. Our people have always had this innate sensibility. This gives rise to the medicine traditions. Where there is humanity there are bodies. Where there are bodies, there is sacred medicine. With both comes boundaries, rules, and guides.

Incest Taboo and Child Protection

In every culture around the world there are strong ethics, morals and behavioural codes associated with gender and sexuality that protect children and under aged individuals. Most models suggest the necessity of the incest taboo as a social value. The incest taboo usually means not having sex with someone in your immediate family, that is, parents, children, siblings, cousins, aunts, uncles… All are included in this taboo. Sometimes innocent exploration between cousins leads to the 'kissing cousin' experience. But overall, the taboo is meant to protect children, youth, and young adults from becoming sexualised. And meant to protect families from the inevitable conflicts and problems that grow from violating these boundaries of respect.

Although we have seen situations where the incest taboo is explored and broken within native and non-native cultures, in my experience these situations tend to be extremely complex and invariably associated with histories of sexual abuse, violation, and trauma. When the incest taboo is violated we tend to see learned patterns of emotional life and behaviour that are maladaptive and dangerous to self and others. Cases may include addiction, drugs, alcohol, and socio-economic hardship. Over time experiences can become behavioural patterns. Then neurologically embedded to form counterproductive beliefs. This is precisely why sexual conduct is such an important area for families to keep sacred and to carefully monitor. We believe every human being has a sacred right to be protected from inappropriate sexual conduct during under aged years.

Childhood and Identity Formation

Childhood and early adulthood may be characterised by age groupings: 0-6 is considered early childhood; 7-13 middle childhood; 14-17 late childhood. In prior models across many cultures 14-17 was considered early adulthood. Legal and cultural frameworks have extended early adulthood to between 18-21, perhaps older.

Childhood involves learning and identity formation along with a growing awareness of body, relations of trust, and learning through sensory experience. Early childhood is not associated with sexual development in healthy children. Sexualisation happens in the presence of confounding factors like childhood sexual abuse that includes premature exposure to sexual realities.

Sexual abuse as a phrase many people misunderstand because abuse is often thought to be physically violent. Sexual abuse includes non-physical exposure to sexualised information as well as witnessing sexualised acts. Sexual abuse includes any form of drawing children into actions or emotions associated with sexual behaviours.

In healthy children and youth, innocent and normal experimentation around body and sensory experiences among peers is quite another thing. This does not need to be, nor is it normally sexualised. A healthy degree of curiosity and limited physical encounters among peers is not uncommon. No degree of adult supervision can totally prevent these experiences. But they can be informed by healthy parenting. This involves giving children protective behaviours.

Protective behaviours include concepts like private verses public. Learning around private places verses public places also helps to understand social and communal boundaries. For example, children can be taught what private body parts not to show to anyone but parents or a doctor. Public body parts anyone can see. For males and females these body parts are rated differently in some ways. By informing children of these norms, kids can talk with parents or a trusted adult who is given the role of mentor. If children have experiences that begin to cross the line, their having someone to talk to and ways to think about the experience give them protective skills that can prevent potential harm.

When sexualised information is outside the family control, children may get the wrong idea, and parents may need to step in and provide correction and guidance. Parents need to be realistic about the fact that this may happen and be prepared to support boundaries and to nurture healthy childhood development. There are now many books and materials, educational videos and learning aids that can assist parents with children dealing with issues of sexuality.

Internet and Social Media

In an era of internet pornography there is a ready access to sexual materials, writings, and imagery that can completely change the playing field for children and youth. Families and communities are struggling with how to maintain strong boundaries of respect with new technologies. Most native communities are now fully engaged with Facebook and other social media. In many ways the free access to social media has provided an environment for discussion, sharing, and learning that never existed for isolated Indigenous communities. Adult monitoring of children and youth on social media is an important responsibility for families.

Over the past few decades people have said that the age for getting involved in sexual activity has gotten younger and younger, to the point where children of four, five, or six years of age are exposed to sexual information and may engage in play activities associated with mimic of adult behaviours. While this may be true, the long-term effects of violation through early childhood sexualisation is poorly understood. Though as therapists we see the results in the lives of adult survivors of childhood sexual abuse, and no one should have to live with these issues throughout their life.

More generally, as therapists we also see how babies and children's often naked or exposed images and the details of under aged people's lives are fully exposed on social media by parents, family, and friends. We question the long-term effects of this exposure on identity development. Rising rates of mental health issues may be associated with these types of exposure among youth. No type of social media is actually private. Because of social media we are seeing the radical loss and redefinition of privacy. And really, at the end of the day, we need to ask ourselves, why post this image? What stress or anxiety are we giving our children in the future when they see this level of exposure? Do we really have the right to present our children's lives in such an exposing and public manner to anyone outside of our immediate family circle? Would we print off this image and walk around our community, giving the image to all the people here, in the next city, and the next country, and around the world?

We can imagine one day children from this era may take parents or schools to court for damage to their safety and identity. There may be a subset of youth and adults who deal with chronic anxiety and stress associated with Internet Violation of Privacy (IVP).

Adult Survivors of Sexual Abuse

Research on adult survivors of childhood sexual abuse suggests there is no doubt that the impact of sexual abuse is grave and leads in many cases to long term adjustment and post-traumatic stress disorders. Ambivalence is a common characteristic of sexual abuse because the experience is confusing for children, and confusing as one gets older and the experience is translated by time and memory. Combining aspects or layers of guilt, shame, pain, and pleasure make sexual encounters doubly confusing for minors and for adults looking back on their early experiences.

Our work with these cases involves adults who enter therapy for long term personal and relational patterns. Many have never shared their early sexual experiences with anyone, having kept these secrets most of their life. Others are more open about the abuse they endured but come into therapy due to relational patterns, inability to maintain intimacy, or broken relationships.

Boundaries around childhood and becoming an adult have much to do with the passage into intimacy and sexual activity. There is a positive developmental purpose to Indigenous initiation ceremonies that provide protective factors, instil respect and other key values, and give youth clear guidelines on social boundaries. This places emotional, spiritual, and physical intimacy into their proper contexts of safety, caring, and consideration.

The passage from youth to young adult is a vitally important time of learning. When one stage of identity moves into another. This provides times for parents and other adults in a young person's world to prepare that young person for the responsibilities of caring for personal safety and for taking care of other people.

Early Adult Initiation

As puberty tends to be around age twelve, initiations into early adulthood traditionally happen during this time or soon thereafter. Historically there is a dual purpose to initiation. One is to help prepare the young person for adult responsibilities. Two is to signal to other people that the youth is becoming an adult, and to provide the young person with support and guidance in the coming years to full adulthood. Several Mi'kmaq Elders have suggested to me that the traditional age for initiation was thirteen. This number is associated with many other ecological, cultural and spiritual teachings. Even the poles of the Wigwam are 13 in number. And they each hold a story and a teaching.

Legal age in modern cultures has moved up to 18 in most cases because this allows five or six more years to adjust to the complexity of adult rules and laws that exist in modern societies. Looking at 13 to 18 as an adjustment stage is helpful. Having protection from sexualisation and abuse is important during these years. Being protected from the many pressures and anxieties that premature intimacy and sexual experience can bring is also important. Providing young adults with greater freedom from adult pressures and responsibilities as well as time to get things right before making these commitments is worthwhile.

In many ways, native cultures see kids growing up very fast. Many are parents before they are out of their childhood mindsets, and a lot of these youth-parents need the help of their parents and grandparents to raise children simply for the fact that they do not have the maturity or skills to raise children yet themselves. In other ways, grandparents who survived residential schools did not receive positive parenting imprints and did not develop the skills necessary to raise strong families. In spite of all these factors, native families are resilient, and people can grow as much through trial and error as we do through ideal circumstances. Overall, people need stability and longevity in their relationships, while perhaps exploring and experimenting where they find space to do so.

Within these stable relations that promote longevity and commitment are many less discussed intimate relations that may occur from time to time. Sexual ethics among native cultures tend overall to be less black and white than in the European-descent cultures. Marriage can more easily be dissolved between consenting adults. Notions of consent hold a great deal of respect. Deceit and hidden agendas are not well tolerated, although they may occur where people have not gained enough integrity or confidence to share their ideas and choices with their close relations.

All the more reasons why early adult initiation into cultural norms is so important and needs to be addressed by Indigenous families. In this day and age, a greater degree of confusion is common because of exposure to broadly liberal social ideas via internet and social media. Making local cultural values clear can be a greater challenge than in past. The same is true around keeping our language alive and well. Sharing cultural traditions over social media are part and parcel of creating spaces for youth to engage and care about their culture.

Drawing Firm Lines in the Sand

In many colonial and Fourth World situations such as in Australia, Canada, the USA and New Zealand, certain Aboriginal people may think that their tradition supports abuse and violence, but this is not true. In virtually all of these cases such beliefs arise from the trauma of colonial violence and oppression. These past experiences of extreme abuse, including outright attempts at genocide result in an internalised trans-generational cycle of trauma. This needs to be addressed through cultural restoration, reconnection, and wholistic Aboriginal methods in spiritual healing. These approaches are proven again and again to restore people's innate sense of dignity and respect for self and others.

Across all Indigenous cultures it is clear that sex with minors constitutes grave sexual misconduct. As a psychotherapist these issues also raise concerns for the adult individual's psychological, emotional and spiritual well-being. And in the case of the minor or child involved, there are on-going concerns for support, therapy and education that are oriented toward establishing and nurturing healthy and clear interpersonal boundaries.

Pathways to establishing safety, clear definitions of personal space, and on-going support throughout childhood may result in a youth who has a fighting chance of normal adult intimacy. Nurturing support systems in families where they have not existed for two or more generations is challenging though not impossible.

Child protection policies often appear to counter efforts towards building strong families. Further dividing families and communities, breaking apart kinship groups, and rendering children and families nearly completely powerless only adds to the prevalence of trans-generational trauma that leads to the decrease of protective factors in families then leading to an increase of incidents of child sexual abuse. Broad native-culture-based collaborative interventions are desperately needed now and in future. How sad to be saying this well into the 21st century, good heavens.

There is no doubt that where families degrade into sexual misconduct and engage in abusive and violent behaviours, the wider community has an ethical, moral and legal obligation to intervene. The circle of intervention may only reach to local families, or to a reserve community for instance, but in very extreme cases the wider Aboriginal society and mainstream society may become involved.

At one stage a myth was being promoted among Aboriginal people, we will not identify the country, where it was being said that men who were violent toward women were carrying out traditional cultural ways. The wider Indigenous community made it more than clear that this was not true and was not to be accepted. They clarified that while traditional culture included aspects of corporal punishment for certain wrong doings, physical and sexual abuse of anyone was not tolerated by the elders.

It is important to realise that these situations of extreme confusion are not uncommon among Forth World contexts where Indigenous people endure extreme circumstances. Every minority tends to engage in self-harming behaviours at one time or other, and this appears to be a part of learned helplessness and of post-trauma. But our focus in life and psychotherapy is on healing ways. We came into this life with an innate feeling for beauty and wisdom. We chose over the years to keep this Medicine strong.

Therefore, our career as a therapist focuses on the generative healing cycle that we observe among Aboriginal, Native, Black American, gay and lesbian, and other minority contexts around the world. In fact, healing is not only possible but desirable. Healing happens. Trans-generational trauma is only resolved through present-generational healing. You can stop the cycles of violence and abuse, trauma, grief, and loss. Yes of course life and crisis and health issues always happen, and too often! But when it comes to emotional, social, and psychological healing from past hurts we humans are actually incredibly gifted. Healing from past hurts can be learned and nurtured. The first step is learning our health-giving ways and unlearning colonial ways. Both path-workings need to happen for us older folks, kind of at the same time, as hard as it might be for us to do two things at once!

Learning Our Ways, Unlearning Colonial Ways

Here we go! Learning cultural empowerment ways is the first step. Mi'kmaq and native ways teach self-regulation, self-empowerment. This happens within family and community. We are one though we are many. Our collective identity is who we are. Empowerment is being part of a people, a family, a nation.

Likewise, learned helplessness is a core concept in colonial studies associated with trauma and healing. The trauma and healing cycle involve internalising violence and aggression while lashing out at the only people available to you - your own family and community. Again, native ways teach the medicine path, ceremony as life, life as ceremony. These methods give mindfulness and heart-focused living. Attention to beauty and right-relations based on respect. This is our way. It is powerful and good.

Naturally there is a lot of anger. Anger over what is happening to our people, our family. Anger over our violation of rights. Anger turned inward becomes either depression or self-harming behaviours. Anger turned inward can become abusive to family members or people in our communities, or also to visitors whose intentions may be pure. Anger among our men can be very damaging because the power of spiritual warriors is misguided into acts of violence or aggression that have no meaning, no real purpose except letting off steam. This can be hurtful, and people end up in hospital or turned away forever.

Better forms of anger-work need to be promoted. Taught. Learned by boys and young men. There is always a choice, even in that second when the fist is raised there is a choice. A choice means power. Acting in rage and anger is giving away your power and being weak. A weak man strikes another. Native warriors learn self-control and purpose in their hunt, in war games, and in times of war. They pray for their enemy with a pure heart, they never lash out in uncontrolled anger even in battle. This would be to give up your power. To be weak and giving into the fear that anger brings. Anger and fear are two spirits that dwell as one, usually together.

To take your anger and frustration into the wider mainstream world would not be tolerated or safe for anyone even though most of the anxiety originates from the historical relationships of your family with the mainstream cultures who invade and dominate the land in past and now. It is unsafe to express protest and frustration in the wider western context. As such, most minority groups including Aboriginal and First Nation tend to engage in self-defeating behaviours when people are spinning in their own wheels without a clear sense of how to organise their energy to make change and address injustice.

The maze is so thick that people do not know how they got to where they are. Trans-generational trauma results in patterns of behaviour that include sexual violence, physical abuse, substance reliance and financial hardship. Self-defeating attitudes self-perpetuate just like positive attitudes tend to generate more good energy. The ironic part of the picture is that inwardly people possess the same inherent power that has its origins in the Original Teachings from the Dreaming and Medicine Traditions. We are powerful beings who can self-define our reality based on our beliefs, attitudes and actions.

In the same way, the Two Spirit Medicine tradition among the Mi'kmaq people is actually a system of powerful medicine including warrior medicine, beliefs, and values that are highly ethical and deeply spiritual. Self-regulation and control are part of this discipline and practice.

There is no mention of loose sexual conduct among true Two Spirit teachings nor in these pages, nor should there be. The tradition is about relationships of honour and respect that are guided by the central values of the Mi'kmaw tradition of 'M'sit No'kama' or All My Relations, which is guided by the principle of right relations with all beings. In this way, the Two Spirit message is one of Sacred Trust that cannot be defiled by the misconduct and profound confusion of certain members of the community or of wider social forces. There is a core truth that cannot be mistaken. This already exists within creation. Creator gives this truth for all to see. No one holds the copyright or governs this truth, and no human dogma can ever contain this wisdom. No church or organisation can claim this for their own. Truth like beauty is simply existing and part of nature. We either get in line, or we mess things up. Both might be beautiful, although humans messing around with the truths of nature might also get us all killed.

When an elder asked me to write a book on Two Spirit ways, she put the questions to me directly – do I stand for protecting children and family relations from sexual misconduct? My answer was a resounding yes! Safety and respect are the beginning and end of everything we do. My work as a counselling psychotherapist, educator and specialist in human sexuality has always included a strong sense of ethics. This is why the ethics of boundaries and human sexual relations forms the first part of this important discussion and is really the heart and soul of Two Spirit ethics.

The reason for this is clear. The Medicine Two Spirit is entrusted to enter into people's personal lives. This is a huge responsibility and cannot be taken lightly. In all reality the medicine tradition requires of a person a great deal of learning, sacrifice, and growth over many years. Medicine Keepers are not easily trusted, they must earn trust over time. So strong ethics are essential. Strong ethics and values guide the Two Spirit path from beginning to end.

Kisiku Sa'qawei Paq'tism leans forward in the wigwam and stokes the coals of the fire and says, 'M'sit No'kama, Ta'ho.'

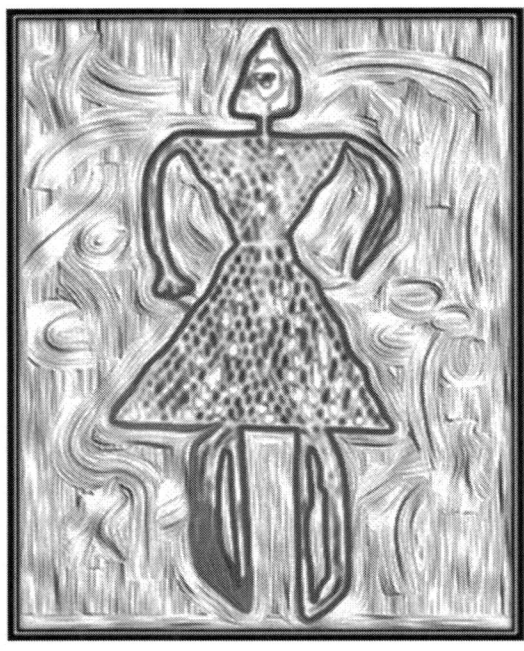

'Sweet Grass is offered to honour these teachings provided today in the Wigwam. We welcome these teachings and offer Thanks to our Ancestors… who have provided these insights that connect with our family wisdom…'

Gender Identity, Gender Variance

Pjila'si, welcome, come in, sit down. Welcome to our sacred fire in this humble wigwam.

In western cultures gender is the key defining concept, whether we are talking about heterosexuality, homosexuality, gay, lesbian, bisexual, transgender, intersex or Two Spirit. This idea is surprising to many and was also difficult for me to understand.

When I first began the professional study of human sexuality, it seemed that who a person has sex with is how people define identity. In gross terms, this is still true. We say you are straight because you have sex with the opposite gender. But does a straight woman have to make love to a male? Well, not really. She can love anyone she chooses. But once she has sex with another women, she might be labelled as bisexual. If her behaviour continued, she may be called a lesbian. Her identity is defined by the gender of who she has sex with.

However, there is a subset of heterosexual people who maintain the added advantages of remaining straight while having sex with their own gender type. These people came to public awareness during the HIV/AIDS crisis of the 1980s and 90s in the form of men who have sex with men but identify as heterosexual. From this time, we know there are women who have sex with women but identify as heterosexual, albeit they come up more rarely in the sexual health literature.

In all these cases sexuality is reduced to defining identity by gender, i.e. the gender of who you have sex with. Sexuality in this dominant culture is hardly an inward and personal territory for self-exploration, growth, and spirituality.

Such is the modern-day conundrum of standards for defining sexual behaviour that codify gender identity into gross material labels. This situation has not been the case during most of western history. But before exploring history we should clarify our opening point.

When you examine labels related to sexual behaviour, without exception they speak to gender. Not only is gender a physical noun, objectified to the sex partner, gender is also a definitive identity construct. Once we move into this mindset, it is very difficult to step away from this approach to defining identity.

A man is defined by his gender. He is not a she. He must remain masculine or fear reprisal. A woman is contrasted to a man, and only recently in western history have women become more self-defining, harkening back to the Middle Ages and beyond when women's roles in western societies were much more diverse and dynamic.

A straight man is defined as such because he is not gay. A gay man is often thought to be less than a real man, and quite the opposite from an upright heterosexual family man. Why gay is the opposite of straight is quite strange. There is actually no clear binary. We might as well say a Granny Smith apple is the opposite of a MacIntosh apple. A straight man is not the opposite of a gay man. Yet English speaking western cultures insist on bolstering heteronormative male ego in spite of how absurd things look. Human sexuality in dominant culture is uniform, much like religion tends to be mono-cultural and monotheistic.

A lesbian woman is somehow a category unto herself, because she is not exactly the opposite of a straight woman. She is more independent, and slightly mysterious to the straight male. She is sexualised and during history has often been demonised, but she also represents notions of feminine power, influence and self-control. Ironically, her gender identity contrasts more to a gay male than to another woman. Her self-confidence and independence are polar opposite to the stereotypes of the gay male as effeminate and a powerless wimp.

Funny enough lesbians add to the mystique of women's power and influence in society. Lesbians can also be mothers, they retain all the primary functions of their gender plus add more. In contrast gay men being the polar opposite of straight men are viewed as impotent, devalued, and as a fundamental threat to masculinity. Or worse, not worthy of mention.

Those who are bisexual today have claimed a separate category that is neither this nor that, and both/and, if you please. Bisexual identity has grown considerably into a subset of minority culture, albeit bisexuals may more correctly be viewed as part of the dynamic nature of mainstream hetero-normative culture with a twist. Either way, one clear sense remains that being bi means crossing over and enjoying both/and, even if not at the same time.

The transgender person feels their gender identity is different from their physical reality. A male stuck in a female's body, or a female stuck in a male's body. In the material world these prisons may feel dreadful and many seek surgery to change the physical gender to match the psycho-spiritual gender. While in older-times the notions of gender variance were associated with cultural and spiritual identity. In this context, learning to live within one's skin-time was considered an essential part of living the transgender path. We can see how having a touch of both older and modern approaches can lead to being happier. The older values provide a spiritual and poetic perspective while the modern physical layers and psychological issues may give a certain degree of clarity and guidance.

The intersex individual is the only identity label associated with having both body parts if not also a blend of both genders in one physical body. However, society never acknowledges that both can exist in one body. Mainstream society demands either/or and often doctors have the right to choose the dominant gender of an infant by doing surgery soon after birth.

But even here, the appearance of dual physical parts would not be a problem if gender was defined in a more fluid manner. Sadly, most intersex babies are cart blanch reassigned by the attending doctor. Many who have grown up this way are speaking out and saying that they would have preferred to remain in their natural state or to make the huge decision about their gender preference later in life. Here again, gender is the defining value that governs human sexuality.

Two Spirit is perhaps one of the rare terms associated with human gender and sexuality studies that is not tied to gender, essentially because the culture in which Two Spirit arises does not necessarily relate to gender in the same ways as western societies. As a dual spiritual concept, Two Spirit speaks to another form of identity that may include varying gendered expressions, perhaps also a third or more accurately an independent (non)gender identity. Nonetheless Two Spirit positions itself quite outside of gender discourse, and for this reason may have the most to say about the phenomenon of gendered identities.

We will first examine the mainstream or colonial frame of reference, their values, beliefs and the resources they bring to bear on their incessant colonial self-made nightmare. From this strategic work we can then appreciate and celebrate our unique cultural and spiritual gifts, values and practices. We can then apply an innovative strategic method and a systematic approach to moving forward.

Analysis of Western Cultures

Notions of gender are complex and very much tied to cultural perspectives. We have only to consider western cultures over the past thirty years to see vast changes in the ways that masculinity and femininity have been defined. The roles of women and men have changed quite dramatically. This process of cultural change can also be seen during historical periods.

For example, during the Middle Ages the roles of men changed from largely farming to taking up commerce in small city-states, seaports, and along trade routes. The change from agrarian lifestyle to commerce, on one hand, led to greater diversity for men in identity. On the other hand, unhinging life from the land led to forms of identity crisis and the increase of aggression and war. Not incidentally, clerical and corporate cultures rose in prominence as a result of independence from Indigenous occupations.

These shifts in economics influenced the roles of women who took up new roles outside of the family home in various types of businesses. Women of high society also shifted in their roles and often took up leadership and had great influence in political matters. At the same time women entered into cloistered monastic communities quite apart from men, gaining a greater independence from male domination. Some of the greatest works of women's literature arose during this period, in large part due to their collective independence from the perceived menial roles they played in everyday life raising children and keeping house.

The separation of women from child rearing responsibility was perhaps the first signs of gendered liberation. We see this as ironic, as woman's liberation is not needed in a culture that highly values women's roles and innate power to choose their own destiny. It is the inherent pathology of the mainstream western culture that defines women's liberation, and to which women must invariably relate in their quest for self-expression. Women today take on male dominant roles of manager and leader in spite of the inherently gendered power dynamics that eat away at a person's soul, precisely because these values undermine authentic respectful relationships.

A culture that devalues women in the first place cannot provide authentic liberation because changing women's roles does not change the dynamics of oppression. Instead what we see is that women simply take on the roles of men. This is not liberation.

The actual work most needed must be to change the underlying values of the culture. Here again, Indigenous cultures provide one of the only sustainable and viable solutions for western people. From a native perspective woman tend to retain freedom to choose their roles and still highly value their domestic and maternal roles within the culture. But native culture has always highly valued women as the first sacred medicine.

During the 17th to 19th centuries, due largely to the lack of centralised government across Europe, a greater diversity of gendered expressions can be seen continuing back into the Dark Ages. But from the 13th century to today, we notice a slow and steady consolidation of male-driven social values that tended to demonise the positive roles of women in leadership, medicine and commerce. The same can be seen for gender variant people particularly gay men, who over time can be seen to stand beneath the status of women during history as the primary objects of demise.

Men who fell outside of normative gender identity became viewed as childish at best, demonic at worst. Where men were caught in sexual acts of pleasure with other men the medieval mind developed the most elaborate methods of torture. Over the centuries many court accounts can be read that detail the accusations and sentences carried out. During certain periods attitudes shifted from tolerance to abuse of power and persecution. During the Inquisition, the Church devised some of the most exotic forms of erotic punishment, torture, and the most painful of death sentences.

However, as surprising as this may be attitudes toward homosexuality waxed and waned significantly over the centuries. Particularly among the elite of society gender variance was highly regarded as a mark of distinction, privilege and personal choice. Europeans saw themselves as the cultural embodiment of Greek and Roman ideals. As such, many men of high regard took on Greek and Roman tendencies to enjoy same gender pleasures as a mark of civil maturity and exercise of power. While the sexual taboo existed for the most part with boys, young men were fair game for older men, and an elite male subculture existed in many European cities dominated by double standards from Christianity and contentious social moralities.

A high degree of decadence and lack of moral fortitude in Christianity preceded the centuries leading up to the great western schism between western Catholic and eastern Orthodox factions. The Great Schism happened from the year 1054 CE. Reading the history before this time is quite fascinating and suggests that the medieval era was in large measure a reactive movement against extremes of sexual and social abuses by the clergy and leadership in societies across Europe.

These social movements led to an historical cycle of extremes between austerity verses decadence and subsequently gave rise to the even more austere attitudes of the protestant reformation. From the 13th century through to the 19th century, science and scholarship grew to become an independent social force and began challenging the status quo. Many of these underlying trends still play large in western cultures today.

Mi'kmaq History and Early Colonial Contexts

When you shift mind set and consider Mi'kmaw people during the 11th to 16th centuries, you see a people invested in developing sustainable and ecological systems of governance. They had an established confederacy across vast territories, systems of trade and commerce, a robust language and culture, and well established civil democratic government. The historical evidence shows their culture to have great knowledge of charting the stars, seasons, and intimate knowledge of fish, animal, bird, and plant life within their region. Their skills of survival in harsh winter conditions are legendary, and their spirituality and culture quite profoundly based in a complex cosmology that included detailed cycles of legends and stories. They not only had an oral tradition but also systems of recording events and forms of writing, as well as the long-time practice of preserving important knowledge in stone carving and petroglyphs.

Back in Europe the Church had been growing to such extremes of power that another great schism occurred leading to the protestant reformation. The splits of cultures divided families and nations, leading to continual war and distress. Powers of kings and queens grew also, while revolutions of basic skills and technologies led to centralised wealth. But growth only went so far before systems became over taxed. The non-sustainable greed of European cultures led to conquest and then expansion into colonies with the sole purpose of feeding the insatiable needs of kings and queens and their elite lords and ladies.

This is why the French came to Mi'kma'ki during the 17th century. But elders remember visitors many centuries before going back to Nordic and Viking sailors who exploited the fishing along the northern coast. Modern evidence supports some of these points of memory.

Wars between French and English led to the demise of French colonial interests, their deportation, and subsequent British rule of the colonies positioned from Fort Halifax. A very bloody history for the Mi'kmaq indeed, let no Halifax citadel tourist guide fool into believing otherwise.

Colonial Gender and Sexuality

The history of sexuality has parallel during the colonial era. In the 16th and 17th centuries, French culture was fairly flexible and more fluid in relation to sexuality and gender expressions. Their interactions with the Mi'kmaq showed latitude and interest in cultural exchange. They were, in many ways, compatriots and kin. This suggests greater cultural affinity that, in spite of the Acadian-Mi'kmaq identity phenomenon, has not actually been studied in any great detail in the English literature. This bears importance for future study of cultural histories. Particularly around gender, sexuality, and Two Spirit studies. Understanding the apparent synergy between French, Mi'kmaq, and then Acadian cultures may provide useful insights.

Once the British came to Halifax colonial power and now familiar dominant gendered roles took over. The 18th century was a time of consolidation of power and abuse of land resources brought back to the Crown.

Moving into the 19th century men who had sex with men came to be viewed as psychologically deviant. Attitudes toward gender and sexual behaviour had shifted toward some of the more predominant Victorian contradictions that still hold great social importance today. For example, the notion of maintaining intensive social discretion while nurturing a passionate private life hidden from view. Taking the moral high ground was important during this time and defending one's honour was an important social display although without the inherent spiritual integrity of earlier times.

During this era medical doctors studied men who had sex with men who were remanded to insane asylums. From their work the field of sexology emerged. Those places of human suffering and clinical examination were, ironically, precisely where the first theories of 'modern' human sexuality developed. The term 'homosexual' first appeared in print in 1869. Only later the word 'heterosexual' emerged in contrast to homosexual. It is one of the more ironic chapters in human gender and sexuality history that heterosexuality was given birth from the concept of homosexuality.

In similar ways, the male elite of the times, like today, tend to presume a role of defining the terms of gender engagement. However, men often fall into their own well-made traps. Male dominated terms of gender engagement tend toward an over simplicity of oppositions, rigidity in demanding social compliance, and the demonization of difference.

Surveillance of these arbitrary norms is then encouraged, and wherever deviance is discovered it tends to be addressed in austere cruelty designed to increase fear within the community. An arbitrary behavioural code of conduct was enforced that targeted any man when they are perceived as weak, inferior, effeminate, affectionate, or simply appeared different from others. In this kind of culture women are generally subverted while any male could become the subject to discrimination.

Colonial Gendered Relations

The differences between French and English gender construction is an interesting point to consider. In fact, this point holds enormous and untapped potential for understanding early colonial history.

It is commonly known regarding the not so subtle gendered differences between French and English cultures. The French have traditionally nurtured a more sensitive and expressive form of masculinity that is more in touch with feeling, emotion and sensuality. The English have tended to view these French ways as effeminate and offensive to proper social conduct. A more in-depth analysis is warranted in relation to how French-Mi'kmaq verses English-Mi'kmaq gendered relations were conducted.

Even in the more astute historical narratives, such as those written by Elder Dr Daniel Paul, there is not an adequate recognition of gender as playing a significant role in social relations, nor is there an analysis of the importance of gendered norms and their impact on European cultural contexts nor in colonial relationships with the Mi'kmaq. By missing a fundamental issue within the social construction of colonial gendered norms, we forget one of the most easily overlooked areas related to present day cultural revival.

Like during the medieval era, men today are seeking to redefine their identity, both in non-native and in native environments. Likewise, by not raising these issues we risk a grave misunderstanding of many of the central issues of colonial relations. From a gendered analysis of history, we can see that English decisions were instituted primarily by men. The construction of gender influenced how the first Governors and their cohorts perceived Mi'kmaw society, and hugely impacted their notions of the noble savage.

It is not surprising that historical analysis has not caught up to gendered deconstruction given these critiques have taken time to filter into Indigenous contexts. Not to mention that this historical development is somewhat counter-intuitive to Mi'kmaq students whose cultural and political values do not align easily to western sexuality and gender studies.

19th Century Mi'kmaq and the Victorian Gender Paradox

In the first pages of this book you will find an historic photograph of an unnamed person of the Rocky Point Mi'kmaq. With great respect we honour this person with traditional Sweet Grass. We acknowledge that this process of honouring our Kin takes many forms, and here in this book we pay respect by discussing the image in the context of traditional Medicine from our contemporary perspectives.

We understand that this image appearing here and the discussion that follows may be painful for certain Mi'kmaw readers. We feel this as well. This image for some reason calls up many of the layers of the colonial invasion. The way this image appears in the colonial office/studio and the way the person is taken out of their home and context, away from family and environment, provides another layer of violence from which we need to heal. Our hope is that the respect we offer and the ways we discuss this image may provide for our young people especially a reflective critique from a postcolonial approach – and an example of postcolonial methods in action to help our nation move forward.

At the same time, all questions aside, we wish to acknowledge that at base we accept the very likely reality that this historical photograph represents a Mi'kmaw person and we pay her our respects. We hope that in some way the process of discussing this image and putting this discussion out there into the community may help this person and her family find peace and strength.

At times, the discussion below uses deconstructive and critical theory tools that may at first feel blunt. However, the questions raised continue the spirit of respect within the postcolonial method. This section discusses the meaning and historical place of this image in our discussion of gender variance within Mi'kmaw culture and spirituality.

The image is used with permission from the Archives and Records Office of Prince Edward Island, Photo ID0000382, 4750/Series 7 (3109/225). The photograph was taken by a well-known commercial photographer Cyrus Lewis of Charlottetown and is part of the Dr V. L. Goodwill collection.

Goodwill was a resident of Charlottetown between the 1890s and the 1920s. The collection includes a number of images believed to be members of the Rocky Point Mi'kmaq, but all are said to be outdoors and around homesteads. The image is unique in being a studio setting. The identity of the person in the photograph is unknown.

Analysis of the image from the Public Archives perspective suggests questions about the identity of the person depicted. Face and hands appear masculine. The staging is deliberate and inflexible. Placement of objects from furs to assorted goods were commonly associated with trade items of the era sold door to door by Mi'kmaq people well into the 20th century.

The image is unclear around the child depicted, it might be a doll, closer digital analysis from my perspective did not clarify this point either way. As such we take the existence of the child at face value.

Contacts familiar with the collection suggest the image is unique and unlike anything else in the collection. This leads researchers who have looked at the image so far to conclude there may be layers of meaning that past analysis failed to uncover. We therefore offer new perspectives.

From our analysis of 19th century European constructions of gender and sexuality, as well as of 'the noble savage' of the Americas as was commonly used, the Lewis photograph is not remarkable. The performativity of the image stands out as overdone in staging and artificial in narrative substance. From the prejudices of the era we may also suggest that the feminine theme of the image may have further resulted in its not receiving attention.

There are however several points that drew our attention to this image. For one, regardless the artificial framing of the pose and the off-putting colonial office, the feminine theme suggests a kind of strength and dignity that comes from this person. At this level we are impressed by her energy and identity, at least at face value. In a traditional cultural sense this might be enough – to stop here and honour this Ancestor with Sweet Grass. In this sense, we do honour in this way, and we have many times. Yet there is more we can explore, and this person's image generously provides a great deal of insight and reflection.

From a Mi'kmaw perspective the person is sitting cross legged. This is generally considered a male behaviour although we cannot be certain how far back this attitude goes. One cultural theory is that women's propriety goes into the deep ancient past arising from underlying values that honour Women's Medicine. Another theory is that more recent history influenced women's behaviour including through the Victorian era, and that colonial styles of dress encouraged notions of propriety. Perhaps the middle of these two extremes might suggest a pragmatic and personal interpretation – how a woman sits is, at least in part, entirely up to her. It is her own how she embodies physical and social comfort.

This being said, some will suggest that a cross legged pose for a woman exposes her in inappropriate ways. If we translate this notion into the 1880s to 1920s the cultural taboos against women sitting in this manner suggest that this woman may have had a masculine quality. Taking this personal preference for sitting in the male pose into a studio formal photograph takes things to another level. Presenting oneself beyond the native community in this manner may have been a bit more unusual. For a native woman to pose alone in a studio is fairly unusual and unlikely of itself.

Given the Mi'kmaw identity is based in family and community relationships, the solitary pose is also unusual. The baby if a real child softens this solitary quality somewhat but also raises questions. Why would a woman come to a studio with her infant and pose in this manner? The infant appears to be sleeping. Where is the rest of the family? Does this person appear in any other photographs surviving from the time?

We have received the question of whether the person in the photograph is female. The question does not convey disrespect, particularly in the Two Spirit context such questions are quite normal and to be expected. Discomfort with such a question raises another question as to why we might feel that way. At some level taking the Two Spirit journey means finding comfort and creativity in the context of gender identity discussions.

If the person is a male dressed as a female from a Mi'kmaw view it has been said that he did a poor job conveying feminine values of propriety and humility. By not sitting leg over leg to one side the male character poorly showed feminine strength, dignity, and power that are common in women's place within the culture. Sitting in the female pose would not have diminished the other gender variant qualities of the person.

However, these statements may take things too far. We might suggest that the blending of feminine and masculine qualities in this person's image, stature, and pose convey strength, self-assurance, and dignity. Many of these qualities we might admire in an older Two Spirit person who has accepted their gender expressions as simply part of who they are.

From today's view we may think that pipe smoking is a male only pastime. But this is not true, and pipe smoking was common for women of the era. The style of this pipe was also common and could be considered a woman's pipe. Men's everyday pipes may have had larger bowls. But again, this came down to personal preference and habit more than gendered pipes per se.

Although the Mi'kmaq had their own cross that predates European contact, with its own cultural associations and meanings, philosophy and practices, the necklace and cross pendant suggests another ambiguity, likely of Christian influence. At another level, based on the idea that this person is in fact Mi'kmaq, the cross suggests an added layer of colonial performativity. A manner of wearing European clothing and Christian pendant suggests a degree of colonial influence that draws a native person to fit into dominant Victorian expectations. On the other hand, perhaps the person was Christian in which case these comments can seem inappropriate. Again, there is a sense of respect where respect is due.

Ash tree baskets woven by Mi'kmaw people were and remain popular and common items. The birch bark canoe is especially decorative and well made. The size of the baskets suggests domestic and feminine use. If the person was in fact the maker of these objects, the image certainly could have been used to promote the sale of native trade items. To the left on the fur rug appears what may be a pointed spear or stick. The placement and purpose of this object is odd considering the careful placement of everything else in the image. We may have thought this could be a walking stick, but unlikely as the size would not support the person's height and weight.

As staged as the image may be nothing here is perfect. The fur is thrown down, objects piled without order, baby blanket bundled naturally without fixing up, child's face quite relaxed or sleeping and natural. The clothing of the person is unremarkable, head, hair, and hat of no particular beauty or preparation for the studio session. Even the place chosen to take the image, on the floor of what appears to be a 19th century colonial office, hallway or sitting room with wainscoting suggests haphazard preparation. We note many images of the era provide subjects with chairs which from the colonial perspective provides a greater degree of dignity and composure. The floor and pose inside a building in particular are again fairly odd for the era.

Taken at face value, whether this image is a male or female, there are distinctly gender variant qualities that cannot be overlooked. The colonial period suggests certain gendered norms of dress and presentation and this image stands out as somewhat out of the ordinary. It appears that the Mi'kmaw person is either a man with feminine leanings, or a woman with masculine qualities.

The question was raised whether this image is of a European person dressed up as Mi'kmaq. From our perspective this image is more likely a Mi'kmaw person. The casual treatment, everyday quality, facial expression, natural awkwardness, do not suggest a cross dressing male. Had such been the case we also suspect the image may have attracted greater exposure, simply by the fact that the male cross dresser's ego would have promoted the image in one way or other. Also, cross dressing images from the era tend to be fairly obvious. This image does not provide the same level of performativity.

This being said, we do note that images of Two Spirit people from other native nations provide a rather natural matter-o- fact kind of feeling. We get this similar quality coming forward from this person from the Rocky Point Mi'kmaq. Though we cannot and may never clearly identify the person's identity unless further information comes to light.

Reactions to this image by Mi'kmaw people today are highly charged because of the colonial pose. For this reason alone, the person can feel very much out of place, apart from country, and separated from culture. There is a great deal of colonial post-trauma that arises in sitting with this image. This too requires respect and healing. Issues associated with the violence of oppression, residential schools, and institutionalisation come to play when looking at this photograph. A great deal of sensitivity in this regard is paid to our Elders past and present.

It may appear a radical question, but could this person be a gender variant and/or Puoinaq individual? Even though posing in an artificial setting that does little justice to their status or identity, is there a Two Spirit quality in this person? To suggest this from a cultural view is quite respectful and sacred. Generally speaking, it seems conceivable that gender variance in some form would appear within the historical photographic record of the Mi'kmaq nation. It also seems plausible that these layers of meaning have not yet been brought into the open. As Dr Paul suggests, this may simply be because no one has asked the questions before or looked upon images with this sensitivity to gender minority expressions of identity.

Thinking from the perspective of a professional photographer of the era, it seems plausible that capturing the unique qualities of the subject was part of their intention. Perhaps they saw what a modern eye might see – there is something a bit out of the ordinary in this person. This image presents a kind of gendered mystery, and this fits well within the respect and honour given to native Two Spirit identity.

It was common of course to provide such images for crass consumption or monetary commission. Especially titillating to the European gaze of the era was the existence of something unusual. Such was the taste for the exotic. If so, this would not be unlike similar images from other tribes of the Americas. But on the whole, the image does not perform well for such consumption as it is simply a bit ordinary. This quality alone endears us to this image as the quality of ordinary diversity seems characteristic of Mi'kmaw dignity and poise.

European Projections of Sodomy, Homophobia, Savages, and Racism

During this period, European values around gender and sexuality had become quite rigid and over burdened by notions of psychopathology. There is mention in the historical records of institutions for pathology where men were remanded for treatment of same sex behaviour. It was common to provide shock therapy, and in more extreme cases lobotomy was recommended. We have wondered whether it may be useful for a future research project to survey remaining records from the era to uncover whether there is mention of Mi'kmaq or Amerindian persons remanded to custody within the mental health systems during the turn of the century.

It is sad how the historic Eurocentric colonial and medicalised prejudices interacted with native cultures in Canada, leading to further missionary expansion and colonial invasions of family, tribe, and culture. The movements of this time would have in large part led to the residential school era that followed, and to which many of our existing Elders have survived. This is another reason why the Rocky Point Mi'kmaq image is incredibly poignant. She represents a very dark time in the nation's history, which in many ways we might prefer to forget. But we will not forget. Challenging the very core of native identity and spirituality is this form of colonialism and its impacts that are so long felt and central to current efforts in survival and revival of language, culture, and spirituality.

Going deeper into history, there are numerous historical records found within the courts of Europe where men were found to engage in behaviours associated with sodomy. Sodomy is the older term used to describe same-gender sexual behaviour.

During my doctoral program I investigated many of these records and came to understand more about how male gender, male sexual behaviour, and Christianity in western European cultures were combined to make the most lethal comorbid mentality. This sociopathic perspective had spread since the late medieval period into every level of European cultures.

The presumptive ethos of male dominance through the Church governed life from the 14th century onwards. By the 16th century increasing signs of homophobic policies and attitudes were in evidence that objectified sexual behaviour, solidified socialist and centralised power in the Church and state, and placed an iron chain around the stratified social order based in patronage and wealth.

By the 17th and 18th centuries the worst of oppressive systems had been well honed by strategies of medieval torture. These translated into state-based legal codes and high levels of social and familial surveillance. By this time homosocial networks had largely gone underground. Ironically the Church clamped down on homosexual relations between clergy, but the reverse psychosis of fear and denial inspired the tactics of the inquisition. Repression of human sexuality turns ugly particularly when combined with religious zeal and militancy. From the 18th and 19th century, cases that appeared in the courts revealed the now often hidden and shamed worlds associated with same gender love, eroticism, and sexual behaviour.

The words gay and lesbian come from a specific Euro-American lineage. This has been clearly traced to 18th and 19th century European and American contexts where social movements of gay and lesbian men and women sought liberation from the oppression of their societies.

The word 'gay' appears in the English language during the 1100s, with origins in Old French, 'gai.' The meaning was associated with being joyful, carefree, bright and showy. With a rather colourful history, by the 1600s the word became associated with immorality. Into the 1700s connotations with carnal pleasures became overt, as well as associations with sexual addictions, prostitution and the 'gay house' or brothel.

Usage in relation to homosexual men appears as early as the 1920s and appears to be used to suggest being carefree and uninhibited. Before this the term was mostly associated with unconstrained heterosexual cultures. It is useful to realise that homophile communities across Europe appeared quite overtly during the mid and late 1800s into the early 1900s up until the great wars of that century.

There is little doubt that the spirit of gender liberation was dampened by war and hardship and was subsequently subjected to systematic genocide by the Hitler regime that targeted gender variant men and forced them to wear a pink triangle that identified them as homosexual. However, many of the origins of the 1960s and 70s gender and sexual revolutions have their beginning during the movements of late 1800s.

From a Mi'kmaw perspective, giving a name calls up honour, a sense of purpose, and place. Identity grows and follows over time. There are qualities of character, social dimensions, and relational meanings. Reflecting in a different way on the history of names like gay and lesbian we can see how these names can come to carry a unique importance in Indigenous cultural contexts.

The social movements of the late 1800s captured reviving and empowering notions for gay men that had been arising throughout the enlightenment era, an idea that western humanity had sidestepped and forgotten. These inspirations came from men and women in Europe who stood against the oppression of others who called them 'homosexual' as a label that meant they were deviant, full of sin, and shameful. Standing within the enlightenment tradition stood against what they viewed as outdated social beliefs, religious based oppression, and they self-named their identity and later their community with the term gay. Within this several commentators suggest early gay men identified more ancient links to pre-Christian cultural origins where gender variance was celebrated.

Two Spirit Contexts

Blackwood (1997) suggested that western models of human sexuality were not adequate to describe or understand native conceptions of place, self, and identity which offer diffuse meanings and deep-interconnecting associations that place sexual practices at the background of social and communal ethics. This approach contrasts the Euro-American emphasis on sexual taxonomies.

Freeing ourselves from neo-colonial domination requires enormous efforts to imagine the world from different cultural spaces (Bishop 2005) where knowledge itself arises from a different process than the dominant (and narrow) approaches of the west that are focused on cognitive and empirical measures. Cultural survival depends on re-writing the narrative (Battiste 1977) from post-colonial perspectives which honour and foreground alternative cultural traditions (Battiste 1998).

Two Spirit means many, many things, and can be said to mean people who carry the spirits or energies of both male and female in one body and in one lifetime (Brown 1997). The term does not mean men, women, lesbian or gay – as these terms arise from a different cultural tradition that conceived of gender and sexuality as two contrasting and opposing forces of human nature. In many native traditions the energies of what we call men and women today were felt to be deeply interconnected and complementary energies that when united provided explosive creative life-energy that sustained the raising of children and the enduring of family, tribe and nation.

In the western anthropological tradition, the term 'berdache' was used to describe European views of gender variant men mostly, although females seen to be acting as males were also included to a lesser degree (Callender & Kochems 1983). Most of European views focus on men and male sexual variance to the exclusion and overlooking of women's experiences, a tell-tale sign of the cultural values that promoted male dominance in the west (Champagne 1997). This contrasts the 'gift of sacred being' that is foregrounded by native spiritualties of communal ethics and morality. Not to idealise the native conceptions, as in any society there are variations and contradictions. Yet the foundations of the native North American Indian way of life demonstrates and still manifests a form of sacred pleasure in ceremonial beauty, form, and movement that characterize the very nature of Two Spirit poetic being. One unique form of being among the many variations of being within creation (Bowers 2007b, 2005, 2005a).

This is a very different story than we find in many communities today. Communities including reserve and off-reserve, status Indian, and non-status Indian, urban and rural, representing many hundreds of thousands of native people in Canada, the USA, and surrounding territories and nations, are all struggling under the weight of being fourth world countries within dominant colonial nation states (Duran & Duran 1995), giving rise to fractured psychologies that manifest the dis-ease and trauma trails of alcoholism, violence, abuse and loss of identity.

Few are the methods that can address these complex issues (Duran 2006), but there are many who are working to heal our nations (Bowers 2010, 2010a, 2008, 2008a, 2007a). Two Spirit children and youth today may grow up in families who carry the prejudice of Euro-American ideas of sexual and gender deviance, shame in being gay, and who define gender and sexuality in dominant contrasting terms between men and women (Chapple & Kippax 1996, Comeau et al 2005).

Traditional methods are rare, and rarer than they ought to be. This is largely due to histories of oppression where traditional teachings including Two Spirit sacred medicine traditions were suppressed under the colonial regime. Traditional became too dangerous and would result in censure, white-violence, loss of children to institutional schools, and loss of means to survival (Cook 2005, Duran 2006, Etter et al 1999). Also, today these cultures of ideas continue in a sense where many assumptions that terms like gay, lesbian and bisexual can easily apply to native cultural spaces, which is at basic levels a false assumption (Garret & Barret 2003). As we have said, these terms carry different histories. Yet they are claimed by native people in unique ways.

Although the western materialistic-based philosophies of gender and sexuality are used by many native people, along with alternative meanings for mainstream terms, it is important for practitioners and educators to understand the history of these terms which arises from western European histories dating back to the 19th century emergence of sexology and the study of human sexual pathology (Foucault 1978).

By uncovering the deeper cultural meanings of terms, we find that Two Spirit is a very different set of values than arising in the terms gay and lesbian. We also come to see that the issues of prejudice found in homophobia and heterosexism is largely a European cultural and spiritual problem that has been transplanted into native communities around the world. Particularly wherever the British Empire has invaded and settled in Aboriginal territories giving rise to increasing issues of youth suicide (Green 1996), gender violence (Griffin 1998), misrepresentation of transgender as deviation from norm (Halberstam 2005), as forms of shameful identity and self-loathing (Kaufman & Raphael 1996), as twisted religious dogma underwritten by gender violence and male-dominance over creation as well as women, elders and youth (Krieger 2002), and as inherently biased forces that diminish self-determination, empowerment, and personal identity (Nadeau & Young 2006).

All of these underlying prejudicial strategies account for approaches to native and Aboriginal relations that give rise to genocide, sustained violence, and systemic prejudice (Neu 2000). At the cultural interface we see very many contradictions that speak to the pathologies of European and British values that are today strongly critiqued as unsustainable methods of human relations with others and with nature (Nakata 2007, Orr 2002).

We see that healing and mental health are central starting points to recovery for minority people who wish to take up the medicine trail toward integrity, justice and freedom to be who Creator made us to be (Nebelkopf & Phillips 2004). We were not the savages, we were subject to a collision of civilizations that deeply impacted us for over 500 years (Paul 2006). But we have maintained our integrity in spite of these experiences.

Two Spirit then is a form of being that, in traditional culture, speaks to ways of carrying the sacred medicines of the elders (Restoule 2000, Roscoe 1998, Stefanson 2009). Walking in a sacred manner for Two Spirit people is to care for the elders, and to offer our talents to family and community freely (St. Pierre & Long Soldier 1995). The value of Two Spirit cannot be separated from that of country – of the land and sea – from which the People receive their Dreaming and Medicine (Strelein 1998, Tree 2004).

While much research focuses on sexual identity (Walters et al 2006) there are also many studies that focus on the cultural, linguistic, and deeper spiritual conceptions of Two Spirit and human gender relations (Walters & Simoni 2002, Walters et al 2001), giving rise to clarity around justice and the politics of identity (Wells 2006, Wilson 1996, Woomara 2006).

This work certainly entertains the need to decolonise the body, to strip away the layers of shame and false propriety to become a naked being in flesh, once again, in the nature of life before social meanings corrupted a sense of self as sacred, given to pleasure, and open to love and being loved (Young & Nadeau 2005). To use a western metaphor, we need to become a sexual sacrament – a form of being that is given as sacred giftedness, spiritual presence, and erotic wonder restored to health, balance and beauty that arises quite apart from issues of fear, shame, or guilt.

Two Spirit expressions can include notions of gay, lesbian, bisexual, transgender and many of the other descriptions arising in contemporary discourse including queer, metro-sexual, and/or inter-sexed. Two Spirit represents a particular cultural tradition aligned with spiritual teachings and responsibilities tied to communal and familial tribal ways of being. We are who we are because of our family, our tribe, our nation.

We are Two Spirit because we are connected with our tribal country and we carry the medicines of this sacred place because we stand with our elders who teach us the traditional ways handed down to us. We come from many nations that have endured much over many years. So, we know that our traditions today are of course different from pre-colonisation. And we also know that what exists today in our teachings arises from real lived experience that carries wisdom as well as ancient underlying values and principles that have endured for likely thousands of years and within certain oral traditions.

Two Spirit beings are a matter of profound pride in many of our elders and leaders – because we Two Spirit carry a unique giftedness of the fullness of natural spirits and energies within creation. By walking between the two worlds we symbolically are said to embody an internal balance that all beings aspire towards. It is important therefore that Two Spirit people also aspire toward a deep abiding sense of integrity, ethics, and moral standing that inspires the rest of the family, tribe and nation toward greater peace and harmony. As Two Spirit people part of our destiny lies in our ability to carry the medicine traditions of our People – to do this requires profound respect, humility, openness to learning, and an internal ability to self-correct and to grow in being.

Stigma as Waning Moon

The stigma against the 'homosexual' was finally broken in the fields of psychology and medicine during the 1970s. After this time, it was no longer thought to be a form of sickness. Science determined that the conclusive evidence supported a healthy lifestyle model of homosexual behaviour. By the 1980s virtually all research into the social deviance and psychopathology of being gay was stopped.

This was the same era when Aboriginal people in Canada and Australia were first allowed to vote, when women moved forward through forms of gender liberation, and when many other forms of western oppression were being overturned. Some commentators suggest that had feminism not emerged within western cultures there would have been a sparrow's chance in hell for the gay and lesbian liberation.

However, gay and lesbian scholars might more convincingly propose that had the homophile movements of the 19th century not sparked waves of critique of gender identity in the first place, that the feminist movements of the 20th century would have been delayed for a considerable period of time. Indeed, feminism takes its first and most powerful fire from marginal spaces within the western psyche. In a similar way that Two Spirit is important to native cultures, gay and lesbian holds a place of power in European families. But this is not widely acknowledged.

Ironically, much like a lot of gay discourse in society is really straight men talking about themselves, the same rings true with feminism. Women's discourses of liberation would not exist apart from the dominant male constructions of masculinity that set the stage for interactions with women. Women define much of their identity in relation to men. Only the more rare and astute women find their space to self-define their identity quite apart from gendered biases.

Since the 1980s research into gender and sexual difference has focused on defining the basic sociological and health issues facing gay, lesbian, bisexual and transgender people. During the 1990s and following the AIDS era, a healthy lifestyle model emerged that now defines the LGBTIQ2S+ discussion. The first decade of the 21st century saw research move into defining notions of homophobia and gender bias. These efforts continue to challenge mainstream approaches to health and wellness, giving food for thought in addressing the bias and prejudice of medical, psychological, and educational professionals.

Current scholarship follows on civic developments on gay marriage and continues with normative theories, i.e. focuses on a healthy lifestyle model of human gender and sexual identity. Research has all but stopped on the question of changing the homosexual into a heterosexual as being gay or lesbian is now considered by western science to be a normal variation within the species. Studies today focus on how same-gender relationships can overcome prejudice, move forward and sustain healthy families, raise children and become more integrated within western society.

Studies will continue along these lines while more innovative work will explore the subtle dimensions of same gender love and lifestyle issues. As Elder Dr Paul suggests in the Foreward, ironically traditional native cultures never really had to deal with these prejudicial questions or concerns. From what we understand about Mi'kmaw attitudes and philosophies it is entirely plausible that gender variance was and remains largely accepted and not an issue per se. Rather native cultures continue to deal with the internalising effects of colonial influences and as such a great deal of detoxification is underway during this time of cultural re-awakening. Certainly, having a 'separate' cultural identity provides alternative perspectives on many issues that mainstream society gets stuck on.

Modern western scholarship by contrast needs to show greater support for gay relationships including marriage and the raising of children. Studies increasingly confirm the adaptive function of human gender and sexual identity, allowing us to see that when people take a balanced and health focused approach, children tend to grow up in even more nurturing and secure social environments.

Research into child and youth gender development suggests that children internalise gendered scripts and externalise these into patterns of behaviour among their peers. When they observe adults engaging in double standards, hiding of information, and negative attitudes toward gender variance and gay relationships, children render these patterns in overt and aggressive social behaviours. They internalise the unresolved and unacknowledged conflict of values that the adults in their world carry around.

Unconsciously children and youth are attempting to resolve these conflicts, but they do not have the tools or level of awareness to achieve this. The prevalence of teenage suicide associated with gender variance and sexuality issues is at least four times higher than the general population. This is considerably higher in First Nations contexts. These issues arise at least in part from these internalised conflicts that emerge as problems in identity. From a 2014 American study Indigenous GLBTIQ2S youth self-harming rates are recently as high as 23%, meaning one in four youth will struggle with these issues. Regardless what sexuality a youth may come to embody, anyone and everyone is subject to the same internal pressures. Many youths find this process too much to carry and simply want to end their anxiety and suffering.

At the same time, internalized colonial beliefs and attitudes are extremely difficult to cleanse from the psyche of a culture. Implied is how behaviour informs belief, and over time becomes part of the 'operating software' of a people. This is why cultural revival is so important, as these movements tend to underwrite new ways of thinking. This renewal work requires very careful and intergenerational healing in the ways we believe and in our attitudes. No doubt the Mi'kmaq identity is evolving and will continue to learn from experience. In many ways this is a work of cultural and familial therapy.

Youth Suicide

Although studies in youth suicide suggest there is actually no clear way to predict what kind of behaviour may lead up to a suicide attempt, there is little doubt that the internalisation of conflicts combined with major social scripts around gender, sexuality, cultural identity, economic hardship, and prospects for the future play a part.

It is important to remember that we are all deeply relational creatures who need authentic, honest and open communication. To share our inner world with each other is actually an incredibly complicated process with all kinds of mishaps and blocks that can prevent transparent and helpful experiences of intimacy. In this context my use of intimacy does not mean sexualised energy. Quite the contrary.

Healthy human intimacy has very little to do with sexual energy. At the best of times adults find it often challenging to share their inner world with each other. Add the inherent pressures of childhood growth and development combined with the youthful emergence of independence and we have a situation that takes a great deal of patience, insight and genuine loving concern.

Native communities today are self-reflecting on what can be changed to help youth to survive and thrive. We have lost too many of our youth to self-harming behaviours and to suicide. It seems to me that the Mi'kmaw elders are well aware that things need to change toward more positive outcomes for youth. One of these areas of concern is gender and sexual identity issues.

We are all aware of how important it is to understand these issues so that we can engage in positive preventative medicine. However, I believe that as much as we are anxious about self-harming behaviours we need to actually create a wider and more positive focus on generating healthy communities while also directly addressing issues of harm and risk.

No doubt that without the contrasting fears and anxieties associated with gender variance during the past, native children need a clear slate to explore and discover their emerging identity within a supportive mind-set. This process will not be easy for some of our communities where the internalised Christian attitudes and beliefs to these issues place the culture several decades behind other native and non-native communities who have enabled a more adaptive belief system. In part the answers rest with moving forward in generational adaptations to beliefs, values and cultural identity. This is a positive process, even for many of our elders. We each have a part to play in reconstructing our collective identity into a more resourceful and empowering reality.

When people come to me for help my approach uses a pragmatic method. My question is 'what beliefs and values are actually resourceful for you?' 'What works for you?' If the belief or value is not resourceful and does not lead to health, freedom, and empowerment, I suggest people change the belief or value. When your belief system is built upon a flexible realistic ecology, you can more easily adapt. This is why traditional native cultural and spiritual ways are so robust and adaptive.

This pragmatic method in culture is very powerful. Native culture adapts by looking at what works. We build on skills and strengths. What worked in past might not work now, so the approach changes. Nothing is more important than creating a world of safety and cultural empowerment.

We acknowledge that Christian religions have not moved forward on these issues, even though there are a few signs of change among some churches. The landscape of social values and opinions on the issue of same-gender love, attraction, and intimacy are contentious. For native cultures this is very slow. Change needs to happen quickly to save our youth.

When Mi'kmaw communities address these issues, the response may be conflict from within and without. The traditional western approach is silence, avoidance, condemnation, and surveillance. Learned helplessness promotes an attitude of allowing others to define the terms of engagement. When faced with inadequate frameworks to understand critical issues like gender, sexual identity, and youth suicide we Mi'kmaq must move more quickly and let go of colonial conflict. We need consensus. We need the Wabanaki way that builds on coalitions and cooperation.

This being said, in my estimation Mi'kmaw culture is profoundly adaptive and always has demonstrated this strength. Kisiku Sa'qawei Paq'tism leans forward in the wigwam and stokes the coals of the fire and says, 'M'sit No'kama, Ta'ho.'

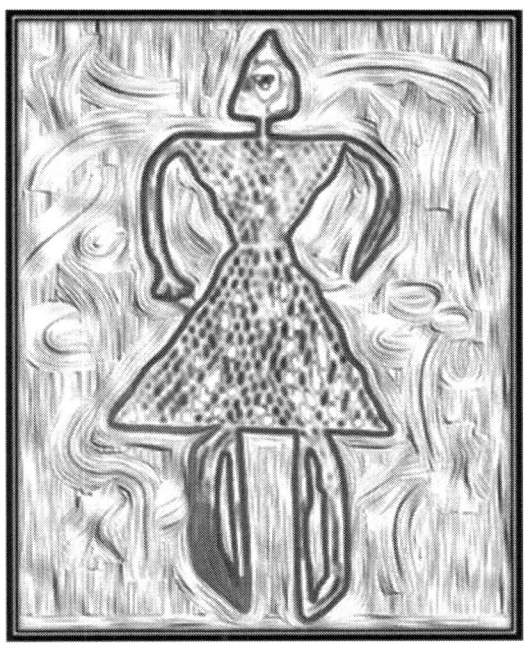

'Particularly now, the current generations are given many tasks to resolve prior conflicts that arose in war, illness and hardship as well as poor choices that led to division, relational breakdown, destruction of the environment, and patterns of anger, violence and abuse which includes substance abuse. We are given these tasks by our Ancestors.'

Two Spirit Ways of Knowing

Pjila'si, welcome, come in, sit down. Welcome to our sacred fire in this humble wigwam.

A number of concepts are introduced in this chapter. Arising from narrative, ethnographic, postcolonial and Indigenous standpoint analysis, we share insights from over two decades of work in the field of Indigenous studies. Two Spirit practice is explored as a cultural and spiritual body of knowledge.

We apply our understanding to assist practitioners who may wish to strengthen their cultural competence in counselling, education and health practice among Two Spirit Aboriginal clients. While this is one focus, we also know that providing this information to Indigenous communities will help families and youth. At the heart is the primacy of personal experience and conscience – nothing can negate the power of an emerging identity built upon resilience and honest exploration. This sometimes elusive yet enduring power within minority persons counters the western colonial and oppressive perspectives that tend to dominate history, social discourse, and that seek to confine, restrain, disqualify, and eliminate the very possibility of being.

Kwe, greetings, in the Mi'kmaq First Nation language. M'sit No'kama, All My Relations. We begin with words from the Mi'kmaw language for symbolic and practical purposes. Initially, to teach the most basic and overlooked necessities of cultural respect that uses phrases from Indigenous languages as an expression of desire to dialogue and grow in understanding of another culture.

At a deeper level, these particular phrases represent a whole field of cultural philosophy comprising the epistemology, ontology and cosmology of a People (Bowers 2010, 2010a). Due to space and time restrictions, this book cannot possibly convey adequately these layers of cultural knowledge. We can only point to their existence and suggest that practitioners take on greater intention to explore and understand cultural traditions within their work with minority clients (Bowers 2007b, 2007c).

We note that 'People' and other significant words in the culture and spirituality of Indigenous nations are capitalized to signify a shift of awareness through acknowledgement of the deep ecology these words convey in the culture (Bowers 2007). 'Indigenous' and 'Aboriginal' are also capitalized to show respect to Indigenous nations, and they are used in a similar manner (although slightly different in the context of postcolonial studies) as the nouns 'Irish' or 'Celtic'.

By foregrounding Indigenous voice, we seek to engage in intercultural dialogue based in greater understanding of the need for decolonizing the self of practitioners (Battiste 1998, 2002a). Such an effort can only proceed with respecting the cultural interface that certainly exists but is too often overlooked in a 'white cultural blindness' that is combined with thick layers of colonial bias, racism and conflated with forms of gendered hegemonic prejudice and intolerance (Bowers 1010, Bowers et al 2010, 2005, 2005a, De Cecco 1990, Fekete 1987, Foucault 1978, Giddens 1991, Griffin G 1998, Halberstam 2005, Nakata 2007, Noel 1994).

This discussion builds on much prior work in minority, GLBTI and Indigenous studies that shows the interwoven nature of bias and prejudice across many cultural, racial, and gendered expressions of difference. To counter the status-quo we propose forms of self-analysis, open-mindedness, and interest in the practice of cultural competence (Arthur & Collins 2010) that arise from this study of Two Spirit identity and practice.

Finding Your Path Through the Mist

For many reasons related to the history and politics of American and Canadian colonial invasion, genocide, subjugation, missionary oppression (Paul 2006), and the parallel minority responses to protect and preserve our Sacred Traditional Teachings through our oral systems of transmission from Old Elders to Young Elders, during the first decade of the 21st century a cultural revival within Indigenous societies has transpired. As part of the 'Fourth World' national context, Indigenous nations exist within colonial nation states. As such, the current pan-national awakening influences and arises from new and public sharing of information from our Sacred Traditions.

Globally much of this information is yet to come to press and is showing its early signs of existing on the world wide web (Stefanson 2009). Although there is indirect evidence of a spiritual tradition specific to alternative genders and sexualities within Australian aboriginal cultures, there are also signs of more open dialogue and publication of information currently arising (Living Black 2009).

The work of Walters et al (2001, 2002), focused in women's health and included Aboriginal participants. In a more recent study (Walters et al 2006) they foreground these experiences to a greater degree, showing the multifaceted and unique cultural perspectives that arise within Indigenous spaces. Their work highlights the need for greater awareness of postcolonial approaches to culture that work to deconstruct mainstream perspectives which are heavily biased by the European traditions of the professions and the academe in North America and in other colonial states.

These ideas have directly impacted our perspectives on Aboriginal concerns. The inherent racist assumptions that exist in non-Indigenous societies within colonial states prevent basic access to ethically competent practice. Across the helping professions these negative outcomes of colonization can be broken down once we understand the mechanisms of prejudice and how they operate (Bowers 2005c). We can then examine how counselling and allied health practitioners deploy these mechanisms in practice (Bowers 2005b). But another key part of the picture is understanding Indigenous cultural experience in its own right, and as having its own integrity. This ought to lead practitioners to engage in cultural competence training that seeks to inform, inspire, challenge bias, and provide tools for sustainable practice.

Assisting this knowledge Brown (1997, 1997a) published a foundational text on the American lesbian and gay phenomenon that tabled some of the earliest scholarly discourse in the field of health and cultural studies. Naturally, earlier anthropological work bears a minor comment in this contemporary context (Callender and Kochems 1983), although extensive revision of that work is required to be of any use in a postcolonial and Indigenous standpoint method that informs a professional ethical approach to practice with minority clients. Champagne (1997) foregrounded the important qualitative notion familiar to counsellors that the client's innate sense of meaning and purpose is 'sacred' business that practitioners need to attend to early in the therapeutic engagement.

In likeness, the notion of Two Spirit suggests a Sacred Aboriginal Tradition that needs to be appreciated even where many Aboriginal clients from First Nation communities may not personally carry a conscious awareness of this Tradition. This level of awareness or lack of insight may have important implications for the level of change or healing accessed by the client within a therapeutic setting. As suggested by Bowers (2007b) during a discussion of a case study montage of an Aboriginal client whose identity issues were confounded by other presenting problems. These needed to be addressed via an integrative and wholistic approach to intercultural therapy (Cortright 1997, Cowan 1992, 1994, Crocker 2005).

We note that the spelling of 'wholistic' arises from a respect for Mi'kmaq First Nation cultural Teachings that place emphasis on working within the whole of analytic, theoretical and practical processes. These principles relate to a deep ecology residing within Indigenous standpoint, coming from the philosophical layers of Aboriginal cosmology (Bowers 2010, 2010a). Within this approach we gain a sense of the Sacred Nature of Story, in this way, 'our Stories are our Medicine.' Aboriginal approaches to social and personal change rely heavily on the cultural place of sharing stories within circles of dialogue, respect, honour, truth, humour, forgiveness, and humility.

Getting beyond the gendered and sexual bias of mainstream beliefs and values is well illustrated by De Cecco's (1990) important work on deconstructing the ways that mainstream values conflate sexual physical acts with identity labels. In this European influenced tradition, 'gay' and 'lesbian' mean, foremost, who you sleep with and what you do with your bodily parts in bed with someone of a specific sexual orientation. There is no inherent moral weight to this assumption that seeks to limit the meaning of identity based on sexual acts.

Likewise, this construct links to a very long social and cultural preoccupation with sex and sexual acts as perverse, immoral, and subject to legal sanction in the west (Foucault 1978). These forms of western prejudice toward sexual difference conflate with colonial culture's notions of hegemonic masculinity, inferior femininity, and these are further intertwined with and define the most basic assumptions around racial superiority tied to hegemonic masculinity (Fekete 1987, Giddens 1991, Griffin D 1998, Halberstam 2005).

To engage authentic encounters in culture we must first decolonize our own bodies and minds (James 1994) and understand that our inherent (unconscious) beliefs and values impact and interact within our therapeutic and educational methods to negatively harm our clients. Likewise, appreciating the complexity of spirituality as a cultural form of how people make their sense of meaning, we also acknowledge that appreciating Two Spirit Tradition within First Nation societies must be a very complex field of study (Jones 2005, Letendre 2002, Roscoe 1998).

There is a growing appreciation within postmodern and postcolonial studies that identity is itself a complex and always evolving phenomenon (Sarup 1996) with changing attitudes toward minority identities arising as mainstream societies 'wake up' to or are confronted by difference (Schwanberg 1990, Sedgwick 1993). There is also a strong and robust acknowledgement in the literature that practitioners across the helping professions internalize the wider social prejudices and that these impact on ethical practice and cause harm to clients (Bowers 2010, 2005b, Smith & Gordon 1998, Plummer 2000, 1999, St. Denis & Hampton 2002, Tompkins 2002, Tucker 1995, Van-de-Ven et al 1996, Watt 1999, Wells 2006, Woorama 2006).

To contextualise Two Spirit cultural perspectives and practices we need to acknowledge the importance of several cultural values including the place of metaphor and story. For example, Bowers (2005a) presents a transformational epoch tale of the 'Shieldwolf' as a metaphor of cultural identity transformation following colonial influences including within trans-generational trauma (Orr 2002, 2002a, Paul 2006). Likewise, the author explores Traditional Medicine practice as a Two Spirit Mi'kmaq individual through a narrative auto-ethnographic journey revealing many layers of cultural and spiritual meaning, including the initiation into the Sacred Role of becoming a Pipe Carrier and Medicine Keeper (Bowers 2008, 2008a). To allow ourselves into this worldview requires we not only deconstruct our cultural bias but also allow creative visioning of a new way of seeing, what a Mi'kmaw collective of scholars have called 'two-eyed seeing' (Hatcher et al 2010).

Expanding these notions, Bowers (2010a) has called this way of knowing a complex ecological and systemic approach that seeks to acknowledge and integrate multi-perspectives across a wide range of practical and philosophical fields of awareness, study, theory, and action. These 'six worlds' represent the integrative and wholistic cultural philosophy of First Nations Peoples and comprise the heart and soul of understanding the Traditional Two Spirit.

Any discussion of Aboriginal methods in education, counselling and health without acknowledgement of the seminal work of Duran (1995, 2006) would do an injustice to the field. His latter book opened up a brave discourse on Indigenous cultural practices within psychology that has sadly been largely overlooked by the mainstream profession. But when taken seriously and within a postcolonial approach to psychotherapy these Indigenous perspectives add to a greater integrity in regard to culturally appropriate practices in psychotherapy. However, we see that for change to happen in mainstream disciplines Indigenous leadership must first articulate standards and guidelines that actually change the discourse, methods, and approaches.

The title of Duran's 2006 work, 'Healing the soul wound' speaks about the volume of work that needs to be undertaken in regard to both the healing of mainstream attitudes, beliefs and values toward Indigenous people plus the very necessary healing work being addressed within Aboriginal communities, families and peoples. Garrett and Barret (2003) offered a useful article on counselling native GLB people, although the basic construct of Two Spirit even within the title of the piece is misrepresented and conflated with the European traditions of gay, lesbian, and bisexual.

Practitioners would benefit by reading the basic and shocking history of colonization itself to gain a more intimate awareness of the weight of oppression and how this is in fact directly linked to what is happening now in our professions. The sustained cultural violence arising from a systematic ignorance never seems to end. This is strongly represented by inadequate and unethical writing, theorization, and professional practices in relation to Aboriginal peoples. Two of the best texts for this purpose are the historical writings of Harris (1990) and Paul (2006). By far the most comprehensive text on issues of cultural competence is the work of Arthur and Collins (2010). Nothing has surpassed this text up to the publication of this book.

A great effort of my scholarly and professional career has been to shift away from 'how to work with Aboriginal people,' towards challenging the dominant narrative. My focus has been twofold. First, there is important work to be done around 'how to challenge and transform the western narrative by applying Indigenous methods.' The second is, from my view, even more important, 'how to apply an Indigenous method of education and therapy that informs services across all applications.'

Turning the narrative away from 'how to work with Aboriginal clients…' towards a revolution in professional discourse in the west that looks at 'how to work within an Aboriginal method and worldview' opens up a whole new possibility for alternative medicine studies within the fields of counselling, education and health (Adams et al 2006, Atkinson et al 2006, Bowers 2010a, Duran 2006, Lacey 1999, Tree 2004, Whitehead 2002). When comparing to other more developed fields of alternative medicine study and practice. Clearly issues of prejudice continue to prevent advancement of Indigenous theory and practice on an equal footing with western models. There is little doubt that the reasons for the slow uptake of these methods rests with the uncomfortable and still oppressive political climate of nations like America, Canada, Australia, and New Zealand.

Where the contentious claims for land and cultural knowledge are ongoing issues the repression of knowledge systems follows within a colonial and political ideology. These decisions may not be universal, but they certainly are part of the decisions made by leadership within education, commerce, and government. These approaches maintain an unjust social order for native people within colonial nation states. A groundswell is desperately needed in order to counter these trends. In spite of the challenges we must move forward in this work of healing so that our therapeutic and cultural communities can begin to exercise respectful and mutually beneficial freedom in the use and practice of Aboriginal Traditional Medicine (St. Pierre & Long Soldier 1995, Strelein 1998, Wells 2006).

Indigenous Standpoint

Indigenous standpoint methods work to critique but also generate new fields of knowledge and practice in research and in professional ways of working (Anguksuar 1997). They propose the deconstruction of cultural bias and prejudice found even within such 'sacred' beliefs of the western academe as the most basic philosophies of humanism, existentialism, and phenomenology that influence the fields of education as well as counselling and health (Battiste 2004, 2002, 2002a, 1998, 1977). Bishop (2005) calls this process the 'freeing of ourselves from neo-colonial domination' in research. Kin with South American liberation theory, this is a powerful turn of phrase when you consider that this challenge actively deconstructs the heart of western methods while seeking a more generative and sustainable approach that works across cultures. These voices from the margins are suggesting that the very ways we practice research and professional methods in clinical practice need to be revised to become more culturally competent (Arthur and Collins 2010). This work, if taken seriously, will in certain ways transform professional practices in the decades ahead not only in relation to minority experiences in education and health, but also in terms of how the mainstream constructs the notions of ethical practice itself.

Bowers, Minichiello and Plummer (2007) proposed in a paper on qualitative research methods in counselling for novice researchers that narrative analysis is a natural outgrowth of clinical counselling reflections dating back to the founders of psychoanalysis, and today related to multicultural uses of narrative and story as natural human expressions of culture and value. Likewise, Bowers (2005) presented a useful framework for how in Indigenous societies stories shared between people with certain intentions are Sacred Medicine Practice and are therefore useful in relation to mind-body healing as well as in understanding how spirituality can be appreciated as a means to reflective healing, change, and psychotherapeutic outcomes.

Holt (2003) suggests that all research engages representation to one degree or other. The extreme of this rests in the status quo in western approaches that seeks to objectify and uses only a strict third person and distant authoritative (and hegemonic paternalistic) voice. Along this spectrum of representation there are many and varied expressions. All of these forms of writing, researching, and publishing suggest in some way the validity or legitimization of what is written and reflected in the writing. Social processes of sharing information and changing of ideas and approaches to any issues arise from this discourse. The power inherent in the research method rests in the ability of people to change their ways of being or acting in light of the research discourse.

Postmodern analysis parallels the movement of post colonialism and seeks to provide alternative visions of value and method (Griffin D 1998). Alongside these approaches the tenor of appreciation for traditional cultural voices stands in solidarity with claims to language, land and cultural survival as well as to ecological sustainability as against governmental, professional, and corporate agendas (Knudtson & Suzuki 1992, Marsden 2010). Also, of influence is the notions of critical social theory arising in post-world-war Europe which have heavily inspired the social democratic movements of Canada and influenced the direction of sociology and social theory in North America and across the western world (Morrow & Brown 1994).

While in my work these notions are not reduced to a Marxian materialism, they are rather parallel to a classical idealism within western theory that acknowledges at least the notion of metaphor, symbol, and poetic meaning in relation to spiritual and cultural perceptions of phenomena. In this way, my method rests in an ontological notion of being as generative, interdependent, and ecological that influences my approach to research and professional practice in as much as I acknowledge the spiritual and cultural as primary locations of how people make their sense of meaning, how they interpret their reality, and how they manifest their energy and intention within processes of change included in healing the self, in creative agency, and in the creation of new forms of matter and lifestyle.

Muncey (2005) proposed that auto-ethnography is a useful tool to describe cultural fields of practice. Nadeau and Young (2006) suggested that these processes ought to help educate bodies for self-determination. In other words, stories self-assist people to see parts of their reality reflected or contrasted or in other ways intuited within story.

Nakata (2007) provided important work on how these methods provide a cultural interface – the place where we actually engage in intercultural dialogue. In the long run of colonial history, this work of supporting Indigenous research has only just begun in fields like counselling where the whole spectrum of theory and practice is largely sewn up by mainstream constructs, textbooks written by white men with grey hair, and taught by professors who presume to know so much about things they know nothing about in reality.

In contrast we take a humble cultural stance and look at the notion of epistemological intimacy central to auto-ethnography (Smith 2005). This sense of intimacy is not only phenomenal to the research experience but is essential and vital in terms of cultural relevance and ethical practice in Aboriginal research-as-learning and as given back to the Indigenous community. Thus, it is important to give back our work to our People, and as such this book is donated to a repository of Aboriginal resources relevant to the People whose lives are enriched by this information.

Cultural Traditions

Two Spirit people within the Mi'kmaq tradition overall have a difficult and often conflicting experience within their families and communities. The Sacred Traditional Ways of the People have been eroded in many ways in many communities. There is still a very strong oral tradition that knows the

Sacred Ways, including the Sacred Two Spirit Teachings, but these Teachings are difficult to access in the everyday world of the Mi'kmaq People today.

Cultural traditions are also alive and well, and stories are told about how the Elders needed to keep safe their Traditions and their Sacred Pipes, and the measures they employed to do so were very often heroic. It is said that during the early days of European invasion it was realized by the Elders of the Nation that the white man would continue to come in strength and would not have the maturity or wisdom to understand the Sacred Ways of the Peoples of North America. They agreed they would hold out in the East to try to slow the tide of invasion for the nations in the west of Mi'kma'ki. In many ways their decision was to sacrifice their lives and wellbeing, and they did for many generations, and have held firm ever since.

Remembering our past discussions of how important in fact the oral traditions are, we need to actually acknowledge that our elders today talk about stories based in 'the great last ice' referring to over 10,000 years ago in tribal memory. Oral accounts of long boats and flouting islands back to what may be the middle ages is nothing in comparison to tribal memory. As a practitioner in western scholarship it is terribly obvious how non-native discourse acts to discount and discredit oral tradition. Yet over decades or centuries now, science and social science proves the relevance of these voices.

However, the key issue here is the status quo disempowerment of native voices for social and political ends that benefit non-native outcomes, followed by many years before being challenged by other mainstream processes that discount the approach that marginalised native authority. But the affirmation always comes too late. This is one of the actual mechanisms of prejudice, which functions to exercise power and authority, literally author-voice, that is always denied to the object of prejudice. We see this dynamic in racism that seeks to diminish the power of native or other racial knowledge. We see the same mechanism active in homophobia. We can therefore examine in great detail the ways these mechanisms were present during the colonial encounter, and how systems of thought and action were used to discredit native authority and voice first by cutting down the leadership and ambassadors of the people.

Speaking again of oral tradition there is memory around an awareness of the deaths and hardship caused in what is now called Newfoundland, and there an oral tradition related to the migration and intermarriage with the Mi'kmaq of Cape Breton Island of many of the claimed extinct People of Newfoundland. The mainstream account does not acknowledge that Mi'kmaq lived on the island. Oral tradition clearly expresses the presence of two peoples who were interrelated without necessarily the same kind of nationalistic lines drawn that European nations tend to create. In fact, we consider ourselves kin with the Inuit further north even if a bit more distant kin. The connections are there and come forward in certain family lines and oral traditions. European accounts make out simplistic notions of tribal identity, and yet the culture speaks about complexity and interwoven confederacies and often intermarriages and exchanges for trade and commerce.

Oral traditions go back a very long way. For instance, I have enjoyed hearing stories of the way the Gulf of St Lawrence was once a small river at the end of the last great winter, the ice age of over 10,000 years ago. The Elders tell tales of how their Ancestors trapped game all the way up to what is now Newfoundland, when all that land was called Mi'kma'ki or Red Dirt Country. Isn't it fascinating? To call this the last great winter implies that tribal memory extends so far back to distant ice ages. In many ways this implication rings quite true, as the elders recall the epochs and eras that extend all the way back to when the land and sea were first formed.

The Kluskap Cycles

The Kluskap / Glooscap cycles include memories that other cultures or modern minds may discount as tales, but in fact they are much more. They arise from oral tradition. Oral tradition is part and parcel of the organic system of scientific methods in Indigenous epistemology. Not literally, not all the time. Yet we take oral tradition into consideration at every turn.

The Indigenous method observes experience and relations within creation, seeking a more complete understanding of nature that can assist people to live a good and happy life. When correctly understood, the lessons and outcomes from this methodology form the basis of teaching and learning, commerce and trade, exploration and discovery, and quite intentional and systematic teachings that guide and direct care and ethics within human ecologies.

Consider for a moment the hidden but also scientific nature of this exchange of energy given gendered meaning, and the ways that gender falls away in significance. Earth being mother receives rays of light and heat from the sun being father, giving birth to springtime and autumn, winter and summer. From two comes four. There is this generativity observed in creation. Families can do this too when a woman receives the energy of a man into herself they together can give life to four seasons. Moon being grandmother provides the light of night, a different source of light from the sun but just as powerful. Two feminine powers and one masculine power, not two gendered powers, but two qualities of nature with three aspects that compliment and complete one another. The distant light of stars also provides another form of masculine and feminine wonder like the expanse of possible worlds, ideas, creation as an act of making new each night. The connection with the stars is very huge in our cosmology. There are few writings that explore the depth and wonder of this fascination within our history. When we pass over it is said we ride the stars back to the place of the Old Ones of the People, back to the Summer Lands.

So, when you consider the poetic or spiritual meaning of natural energies of sun, earth, moon, and stars you have four entities or origins of being and creative power. Do you have males or females? No. Not really. To form a gendered binary is foreign to Mi'kmaw cosmologies. Getting ourselves out of that dominant binary way of thinking needs the most enduring forms of dance and laughter and continual efforts at visioning reality for what reality really is – creative and diverse and nothing at all to do with male and female per se.

Two Spirit people were felt to be Sacred among the Mi'kmaq during Traditional times and are also felt to be this way today, when a Two Spirit awakens to their Medicine, they are celebrated among the Traditional Keepers. Why Sacred? Because the Two Spirit is felt to embody spirits of power, hence the name. Male and Female are not just material genders like in the European way. Male and Female are Spiritual Powers or Entities within Creation, given by the Spirit of Creator, to engage in the Manifest Powers of the People and of humanity. In other words, these Spiritual Powers are qualities of the Dreaming and Medicine of Creation that link us in a familial manner with all creatures and within the life of the planet who is Mother, and the sun who is Father, and the moon who is Grandmother.

The Switch Dance

In the Mi'kmaw switch dance that is taught to children we see how females and males can be encouraged to switch roles and ways of dressing and to take on the qualities and insights of the other gender (Dutcher 2014). This experience provides a person with a bit more flexibility. Much of the problems that come from partners in marriage therapy arise from inflexible thinking. Growing in capacity to dance in the other person's way of being might go a long way to helping marriages survive.

We are linked together in familial bonds with all of Creation. The penetrating rays of the Sun give life to the Seed of the Mother, Earth springs forth with sustainable harvest and abundance. Moon like our Grandmothers guide and temper this growth by providing seasons and cycles that govern the Sacred Law of the Land and People. We are intimately connected with the stars that are the Pathway of the Ancestors. The whole cosmology brings together an integrative philosophy and spirituality, which makes up the organic and often scientific/observational method of the Indigenous cultural way.

Within this culture the Two Spirit person can be male or female, and sometimes may be intersexed (having the body parts of both). Two Spirits may also be more or less transgendered, and some may also yearn to change their bodies into the gender their spiritual being wishes to manifest. However, there is already a deeply spiritual tradition within the native culture that what we are physically given by Creator we can respect and enjoy. While some may still wish and need to change their bodies to be more in tune with their spiritual identity, in a sense there is more fluidity and flexibility to 'shape shift' within the Mi'kmaq Traditional Way. Male can become Female. Female can become Male. People can be of Two Legged, Four Legged, Winged, Finned, or of Leafy variety – all Nations of Creation are family. Therefore, in vision and in some ways in this reality of being, a Two Spirit can be of Totemic Power.

Transformation is inherent within the spiritual energy of being itself. Identity is not necessitated by physically blunt and obtuse reality. Identity is poetic, fluid, and part of the flux within nature.

The physical is merely a passing phase of the ever-existing spiritual reality of the cosmos – we are called in and out of being according to the manifest will of Creation – and we participate in this Two-Legged experience as one small part of the Cosmic Dreaming that is always unfolding and expanding. This sense of Traditional identity expresses the very nature of the Two Spirit non-identity which is not tied to the material forms that European culture worships and holds as their only possible reality. Aboriginal people who know that the depth of maturity in their Tradition often perceives the popular European way of thinking as fairly childish and self-centred, precisely because the material path that separates reality and dominates nature is limiting, fragmented, linear, and flatland.

Likewise, as we have seen the Two Spirit person is not in the Traditional sense gay, lesbian, or bisexual. These European terms do not really apply. However, we can say that a Two Spirit person may also identify as gay, lesbian, or bisexual, as a further way of defining their material sexual identity. For many of us these terms help and are part of healing, growth, self-awareness, and building stronger relationships. From a Mi'kmaw perspective we can fairly easily render these terms sacred, when we take them into the sacred circle of our personal, social, and ecological reality.

From Confusion to Sacred Ecology

In many respects, terms of identity are confused in Mi'kmaw everyday culture. Very few people understand what Two Spirit means, and understandings flux and change over time. Likewise, people can be confused about the use of and meaning of gay and lesbian. After you study a bit of western sexuality and gendered history it becomes clear how these terms are deeply European and American in scope.

Two Spirits who are asked by their Elders to carry the Sacred Medicines including the Sacred Pipe are given many Teachings, and sometimes can be taken into both/either of Men's Medicine and/or Women's Medicine. There is a suggestion in these Teachings that when a Two Spirit person matures into their Power they may come to carry the Sacred business of Men and Women and can contribute a great deal to the health and wellbeing of the People through sharing their Knowledge and Power through their work and their Ceremonial roles. While much of modern writing or scholarship has examined the critique of western and colonial realities and has explored to a certain degree Mi'kmaw social and health issues among the Two Spirit, few publications have articulated the deeper and more detailed expressions of Two Spirit Medicine traditions and practices. There is a sense that academic, scholarly, and professional discourse has not caught on to the fact that these bodies of knowledge exist and are part of the deep ecology, and deep spiritual life of the people.

For example, Two Spirit people in male bodies often come to be taken into Women's Medicine. They may be shown the Traditional teachings, and they may come to help the women and women Elders in carrying their Sacred Bundle. Likewise, Two Spirit people in female bodies may be taken into Male Medicine. Although, some say that the Female Medicine of the People is more powerful, and many men agree, but not all hold to this teaching. We reflect over many years of sitting under the stars that more or less power is illusory and a confused perspective on men's and women's business.

The real issue is not power but how the deep sacred ecology of Mi'kmaw cosmology identifies, observes, and acknowledges the phenomenon of feminine-type energy that is generative, life-giving, sustaining, nurturing, transformational, radical as in deep-rooted, and radical as in causing dramatic change. At the same time, masculine-type energy within creation's song provides a quickening heartbeat, pulse, dynamic, and explosive awareness that gives of itself constantly in service to the primary work of creation as a continual process. To talk about men verses women and sacred traditional knowledge is kind of funny, as everyone can get in on the joke. But to open the incredibly sacred space of deep ecology takes the conversation into an entirely different realm.

This chapter highlights a strengths-based approach to minority practice that seeks to build cultural resources for clients while informing helpers of ways forward. The advantage of this method rests with helpers understanding their roles as cultural advocates, as brothers and sisters to Indigenous people, who can assist in sharing cultural information and in pointing clients to this information when necessary.

Many clients will not be aware of these resources. Two Spirit studies is just beginning. Much relies on Two Spirit people speak up and publishing their perspectives. These practices may begin to break down the barriers that are faced by young Two Spirits who are isolated in their communities. By standing up and being counted as role models, community will have the best resource of all - the value of years of experience and knowledge.

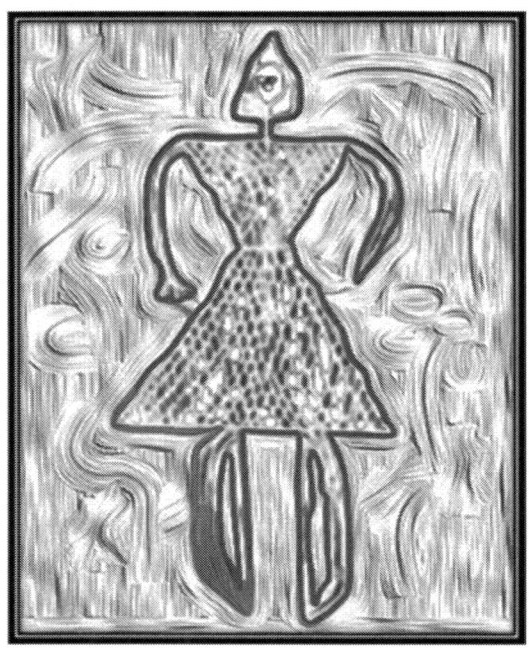

'All modern sciences pay tribute to Indigenous science, because all knowledge and wisdom arises from right observation. When people fail to observe life correctly, that twisted perception leads to harm. Mother Earth has her own logic, patterns, cycles and teachings that lead our People to health and good things.'

Two Spirit Ceremony as Life

Kwe, greetings, and welcome to this sharing of insight around the Sacred Fire. If you lean forward a bit closer, you will see the flames in this fire are turning slightly orange and yellow. These are the colours of youth and of hope. If you look long enough, you may see yourself reflected there…

The reality is that all youth have an innate potential for original and critical thinking throughout their teenage years, and if they were better prepared, they could be doing graduate and postgraduate level work when they hit 20s. But looking at this more widely, all people have the potential for growth and empowerment to manifest original ideas and to bring forward creative solutions to social, environmental, business and cultural problems that we all face from time to time.

The spirit of these insights gives me a profound reason to write this book. This comes from a deep belief that people have within them already the tools for success. We only need a bit of encouragement to unlock our potential. The rest is up to each person. And I also know that when people are offered a way to fall into their own well-being and success, unless they are overburdened by a dead head brain washing from their schooling, or overwhelmed by past trauma and fatigue, most people will grasp onto what makes them feel better and powerful. We are built to grow and thrive. This is the spirit of humanity that I admire and wish to nurture by sharing these teachings.

What we have learned is that each mistake asks us to listen a bit more, open heart a bit more, and let go of bitterness, fear, anxiety or sadness that much more. At every turn, lessons come that impact the way we see the world. These challenges change perspective and give more choices and more awareness of the meaning of human life and our purpose on this planet. The very way we learn has become the central most important adventure of life. Learning is in many ways the same as healing. What modern psychology tends to forget is that every challenge equals an opportunity. When we look more at the opportunity within the challenge, we cannot help but shift our perspective. We are human questions waiting for a solution. The real excitement comes from living in the questions and resting when you need to rest.

Every problem contains the mystery of its own resolution. Every question is the seed of its own answers. All answers generate more questions. This is the nature of energy in this universe. Why? Because all energy is a circle. This reminds me of Whitehead (1988, p. 6) when she described the Puoinaq use of the cycles of life to gain insight. She said, the 'Micmac [sic] shamans, the Puoinaq, prepared for their rituals by erecting outside their tents a tree, a pole, or a branch, often decorated or hung with gifts. This was an outward and visible manifestation of the World Tree…' In many traditions the world tree is a circular and two-way passage through which the seer could journey from place to place. Not only in linear journey but also across many realms.

Whitehead (1988, p. 6) goes on to say, 'As healer and diviner, a shaman of the People often needed to seek answers and Powers in all the six worlds…' As described elsewhere, the Six Worlds of the Mi'kmaq are places that the healer seer could journey. Not so much mythical or metaphorical places but in the old way of thinking actual locations within the observed cosmos. There was a sense in Mi'kmaw culture of scientific or objective observation alongside metaphorical associations and multilayered meanings, such that every story held numerous interpretations. By repeating the techniques of shamanic journey, the modern day Mi'kmaw student of the cosmos, as it were, can relearn and experience similar observations. The ways we might describe what we know will invariably follow modern constructs but may parallel past expressions.

This cycle we call human growth and empowerment rests on the back of problems, challenges, and crisis. Without stress we would all be dead head jelly without any vitality! But I love jelly! LOL! Without the problems that define and build our identity and character, we would all be less than who we are. And we would never reach any potential without being challenged.

But we need not compete with each other. Our inner personhood contains enough challenges for all of us to handle, and we ought to support and be like mentors, guides, life-coaches, and inspiring elders to each other to spur each other on to goodness and beauty. Every achievement of our personal life can bear huge celebration. If we took a positive approach to our everyday life society and family would be so much easier to cope with.

The reality is that our own mindset is the biggest part of the picture that raises the most challenges for our lives, for society, and for family life. People co-create their own misery. People write policies that oppress other people. People create society to suite ease of efficiency but even this attempt tends to fail. Traffic systems get piled up. Costs of living increase. Taxes generate social income but are abused by government. Social rules govern every inch of life, and people yearn for freedom or continue to be dead heads as they were taught to be in state run schools. They buy their socially sanctioned dead head anti-sacred medicine that we call a television, or a computer and they sit for the next thirty or forty years in front of that electronic spirit of domination and control. Before they know it, their lives are spent, and they have done exactly what the big brother forces of society have desired right from the beginning.

How we think is the first step in coming to terms with what we wish to live and how we then manifest that inner voice in the ways of our lives, our families, our culture and our identity. From these levels of living the human spirit manifests changes in the world. We build within the material and real worlds our inner visions. We are creative spirits having a human experience. To grasp the importance of this insight is the central most important teaching of our time. Without harping on this fact, allow us to start into this journey of discovery.

Trauma and Healing Methods

In stepwise manner, here is a process you can test for yourself. Reflect on a negative experience you had in past. In the now of that experience, something happened to you and within you. Lightening is symbolic of things that happen to us that crash into our world, and impact us deeply. In that moment immediate responses were sparked in your body-mind. At one level you may have been thrown into shock. At another level you quickly tried to sort what was actually happening. In one way or other, let's say that some understanding came about immediately, and some experience of misunderstanding also happened.

Many people come into therapy or into sacred medicine work to sort things that happened in the past. Always there are bits of understanding and misunderstanding. The latter is tricky to call misunderstanding. We use the word symbolically. For example, some folks form an impression that stays with them. That leads to all sorts of responses down the track.

Like one person developed a phobia of driving on the highway, associated with the place where an argument happened with a partner many years before. Another person took on OCD traits from childhood trauma. They developed forms of control in relationships that kept the person safe, but also extremely lonely and unable to make connections. Whatever the case, something happened to you. You had an immediate reaction. You had some shock. You immediately started sorting what is going on. And you formed immediate ideas or understandings and misunderstandings. The point is that this process is natural.

You had your dad tell you he thought you were a wimp. You were age 10 at the time. He might have been joking. He may have been frustrated and disappointed. But you were a Two Spirit child and your father saw how you did not fit into your peer group and his expectations for you. The comment threw your little child self into shock and horror. You recoiled inside yourself. You remember the moment as being pivotal and for years after you never felt free to love people in open and trusting ways. While the story and the experience are actually terrible because who of us would want this to happen to a child of ten years old, the dynamics of response and forming an idea or understanding and misunderstanding remain similar for all people.

Now, the inner circle of the self that is formed and impacted by an experience. An outer circle is the layer effect from the experience – we almost grow a layer around our heart when we have a negative experience. First shock protects the inner circle. Then our forming an idea of what is happening creates an interpretive frame around our mind-body.

When the next negative thing happens, we are a bit prepared. At one level body-mind gives us strength in this. At another level, what we learn back then keeps us safe then and after. Thus, we have in that new unpleasant moment feelings of discomfort, hurt, rejection – shielding the self and creating a protect mode. Immediate unconscious layers now kick in. Memories from the past also come to play as our body-mind sorts a new negative experience. Even children do this unconsciously. Often things are sorted in play, games, and symbols.

Then there is an overarching top or rainbow that forms in the self. The shelter is formed inwardly and helps us cope. Chronic stress and trauma form in a person survival and coping mechanisms that protect against our system shutting down. They are positive stress responses in this sense, but over the longer-term chronic stress responses can backfire. What we learn in this process is that in future, say ten years later, the unconscious learned pattern of response and self-protection can often backfire. We will explain why as we go.

The immediate experience in the present moment now connects with over-shadowing from past memories and feelings. Past experiences link-in immediately with new ones. Even though a new moment is happening it can feel that we are being hurt in the same or very similar ways to the past. These are all or mostly unconscious patterns that are operating in the now with all the standard inner voices playing that reinforce the feelings of discomfort, hurt, rejection and/or other feelings that cluster around the historical pattern of response. At one level this is highly normal and valuable. Self-protection is necessary and good. At another level, we need and want to grow, to have a new experience untainted by past trauma.

This is how our patterns have become neurological pathways in our body-mind, when we cannot seem to break out beyond what feel like boxes and barriers and walls. While completely normal this process can kind of suck big time, especially at that stage when people have more or less processed their past negative experiences and genuinely want to grow. As amazing as this seems, this unconscious process is happening to all of us because this is how the human mind and emotional body works. The patterns continue until there is an innate and also unconscious-level resolution to the conflict or basic need.

The immediate experience or process now connects with unconscious past layers. Remaining unaware of this process gives us less choices of how to respond. Becoming aware of the process gives us more choices and we can help to inform, and meet our inner needs, in more creative ways. Feeling ignored & rejected by your mother or father growing up. Getting hit around. Hiding in a shell, a box. Or lashing out in anger, when at the core just needing to feel appreciated or understood. As an adult this process has its manifestations.

Years of emotional turmoil. Isolation. Feeling like you did not belong. Feeling not right. Being rejected by peers. Considering suicide. Feeling depressed and out of sorts. You can learn the skills to step out of this shadow world. It is now important to take a deep breath… In fact, you know what? What we are describing is actually a form of ceremonial experience. But the energy of the shadow ceremony is not positive. The energy is or can lead to self-defeating and negative outcomes for us and for those we love.

The box is not a pleasant process internally. This is an important insight because as you have read in this book so far, you must be aware of the powerful positive self-healing energy of embracing life and meaning and hope. But in all reality no one bothers to explain how to activate this healing process. In truth, it is a skill we can learn through these methods. This is an extremely well-kept secret that needs to be shared.

Think back over this ceremony. First there is a sacred lightning bolt. Remember Kluskap? My goodness... He was hit three times in a row. He was also in shock and dismay! It did not happen immediately, but over time he moved and grew and changed into a new being of power. The Two Spirit path is the same. Racial prejudice is similar. Homophobia as well. What did he do then? He stretched his body out all the way across Mi'kma'ki in the form of what? He stretched out in the form of the sacred circle. His inner self formed new ways of knowing. Wow. This is really true you know, because we have seen this happen right before our eyes. People awaken in this way. It happens all the time. The circle is a growing adult identity.

What happened next? The ceremony of the circle draws him back to who? His nephew, his sister, his grandmother. He was pulled back into the rainbow of family life. This is normalising for us when we have a negative or powerful insightful positive experience too. This is the overarching protective space. The place of ceremony-in-life. Just as the box of trauma is real, so is the box of strength. If you think about this, a box is made up of all sides bound together. It is really a form of the sacred circle with the roundedness cut off. A box is a very strong manifestation of cardinal directions brought into material or psychic form. Self-protective mechanisms that keep a person isolated within their being and in their relationships.

But also, while powerful and strong a box can be self-destructive when inflexible. A box can prevent personal choices and options to grow and change. But a box can also become a safe harbor during a storm, and a place to rest the winter. Do not be too harsh to judge the boxes that people live within, as these places may just as easily be their refuge and all they have to keep things together. What this means is that the box is incredibly strong. This is why boxes are used to send packages across Canada post! Nothing else can survive!

OK now, remembering again the negative experience. You may now connect the power ceremony with the negative experience of memory. When this happens for people they go, this is strange... I can't pull in this negative feeling in the same way anymore. It has changed somehow. Even a bit is important. Now you know that therapy, ceremony, learning, can actually work for you. You don't need a book to tell you. You know.

For Native, Two Spirit, and other minority people with trauma memories, the immediate experience may include unconscious connections with late childhood and early childhood layers of trauma. Feeling abandoned. Lost. Forgotten. Alone. Fearful. Afraid. When I needed them the most, they were not there for me! But recalling this now in this sacred ceremonial learning experience, the flip side is that something new is happening. We don't need to name it yet. Just let it be.

The immediate experience now connects with unconscious connections with still deeper early childhood and pre-conscious memory from infancy. When we go back, we usually actually gain more resources to carry with us into healing and working in change. The circle now feels a bit like a life-giving egg. There is potential for new birthing when we actively learn skills to heal and recover our self. The immediate experience now and unconscious connection to deep emotional and psychic patterns can connect with our ceremonial learning. We are spirits having a human experience. Connecting with this power of spirit is something innate in us but is also a way of reaching beyond ourselves to a higher place that is funny enough hidden in early fearful childhood and infancy states that can be called up in deep memory.

Adult memory of early childhood and infancy patterns of survival. A sense of desperation, existential base-anxiety, terror, fear, seeking connection, reaching out, feeling love, being held by mother, being in the womb… I am OK. I am OK. We must fix this problem. We must relieve this pain. I am hungry! I am wet! I am sick! I cannot breathe! I am lonely! Hold me! I am OK. I am OK. Most processes and memory connections stop here, at this diffuse invisible line. For those who move beyond this unconscious process into the light of awareness the conscious learning or healing process continues.

It easily continues when we have this teaching and ceremonial space of respect for our family, for Mother Earth, for our Elders and Ancestors. We can move beyond even the womb to older sensations and memories that arise in previous times. We have witnessed this in many cases. Healing is forever a dynamic and learning process. Our world is still a place of mystery and wonder. In this ceremonial learning space, you come to terms with your negative and your positive experience. You find they often balance each other out. You can then have more choice of how to move forward. You can more easily consider your goals and relationships. You can influence your relations with people, places, and nature in new ways. Ceremony-in-life gives you new resources.

Sometimes in this space forgiveness awakens. You realise you will never forget, but you can forgive and kind of let go. You will always hold on to the memory and learning, and you will protect yourself and your loved ones in any way possible. But yeah, you awaken to a new strength and power. Being yourself is OK. Indigenous philosophy and spirituality suggest that all life-patterns are inter-connected. Life does not suddenly appear from no-where. Life is a cycle, a process, always transforming. Breakthrough into new awareness is a re-birthing experience. Awakening. Sometimes I think Two Spirit means being reborn twice in one lifetime. Like falling in love two times with the same person. Two Spirit calls us often to die to self, to let go of so much and to be free of cultures and ways that our families and communities take for granted and never question. But we question everything. We leave no stone unturned.

Death as Passage and Growth

Two Spirit is being a keeper of death, a person who cares for the dead. This is a pathwork that many do not appreciate or understand. We help spirits to pass over, just as the ancient poem and Song Line teaches. We are often drawn to the cemetery to visit the graves and take care of our passed. We carry memory of our Ancestors close to our awareness. They often break into our daily life. They bring us messages and teachings. They help us when we are helping other people in healing.

Someone we know takes great pride in recalling the fallen soldiers, and always goes to Remembrance Day events. That person does not identify as Two Spirit. Yet they are a Keeper of the Dead, and they walk with the Sacred Pipe. To me they are Two Spirit in nature, it is simply part of how they walk. Death and life are two sides of one coin. Death is not far from us, not really. Just another passage across the river. We help others cross over. We are like St Christopher who carries the Christ child across the stream.

Like Kluskap who carried his nephew through the deep forest when he was lost and afraid. Like the Great Bear who flies across the Milky Way, carrying us to the Summer Lands.

Once you carry this medicine of Two Spirit awakening, when someone in the family needs help you are there. People see your gifts and you don't need to say much. They call things out of you that were not visible before. Memories are funny things. Sometimes they break into areas that are surprising. Others breakthrough into pre-birth experience & memories of choosing their parents, choosing their life-time lessons. This awareness and this place of being conscious and choosing difficult life-lessons, transforms a sense of powerlessness into a sense of empowerment – if I chose this lifetime to learn these lessons, what am I learning now?

Even if you have not had this experience the idea that you chose this lifetime is something to ponder. It changes the whole thing. You are no longer a victim being manipulated. You are a spirit who chose this lesson, and this means you have a responsibility to learn the lesson and do something about it. When piecing the puzzle together you may realise that native spirituality teaches much about death, loss and grief. These are processes of transformation, changing of form and function. They are deep shifts in identity, which never quite stays the same for long. Growth leads to conflicts, and these result in resolutions. These cycles exist in nature. We native people observe these cycles and come to terms with them over the years.

These insights form a kind of Indigenous ecology, what some may call a theology or theosophy. The latter is more about philosophical models that include a sense of the divine or spiritual nature of things. We observe that Creator appears to provide for transitions and changes in what we call death or passage between forms of energy. Nothing appears to be lost in nature. One thing becomes something new, or reverts to an older form, and is recycled. Energy is always moving and changing. These conscious awakenings help us to look at the unconscious connections, our trauma story, and to put all of that into a new light of awareness, of conscious choice. Awakening. This is really Two Spirit wisdom. It is universal human wisdom and therapeutic. But yes, this is uniquely arising from Two Spirit Medicine. This is what our Elders talk about when they suggest we 'Carry Our Medicine Bundle.' We can only walk this Way when we are conscious and responsible. When we can observe our inner unconscious process and learn to be free to choose our Way with integrity, honour, justice, fairness, patience, love, compassion and truth. Awakening. In every moment. Ceremony is life. Life is ceremony.

Medicine Sacred Circle as Science and Life

The last layer of this sharing will look at the medicine circle. Many say this is a medicine wheel. But wheels were invented by someone else, I am not sure who. Circles rather are definitely important to Mi'kmaw people, including many other geometric shapes. The image used in each chapter of this book is the ancient Mi'kmaq triangle person once carved upon the stones of rocks. We like to see this as a triangle Two Spirit. It could be anyone and everyone. Long before this image was known to me, in my childhood these shapes were drawn, from where, we have no idea. When the Mi'kmaw image was shown to me my jaw hit the floor. Come home! Come play with me! Our circle includes the four cardinal directions or what we call the Doorway to each realm. Each direction in the Mi'kmaq way holds Spirit helpers who guard and teach from that Sacred Door.

North

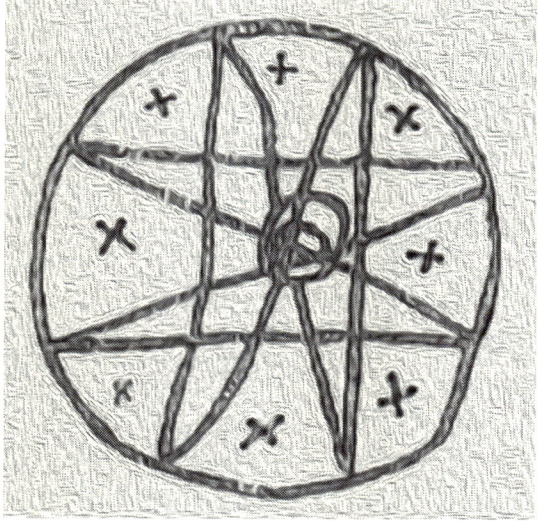

West   **East**

South

You can associate the cardinal directions with actual places and landforms. They relate to the powers of these places, where you are doing sacred business. Not only the local places but regional and global connections. Also, totemic spirits. What many people overlook is the dynamic and power of Two Spirit meanings and connections, awareness comes as personal but also there are layers or connection to Two Spirit powers. These change the nature of ceremonial workings by giving unique perspectives and gifts to the nation, to the family, when we carry these medicines with respect and loving honour. Likewise, what is overlooked today in the rush for pan-global Indigenous assumptions is also that a Men's Business ceremonial knowledge is really quite powerful and unique. There are different ceremonies, song lines, teachings, gifts, and responsibilities that men carry in traditional medicine and dreaming.

The same is true of Woman's Business. And likewise, family groups and tribal associations can actually give rise to quite specific Song Lines and ceremonial traditions. In these ways it is important to learn about your connections, they may surprise you. They often come up spontaneously. And when they are lost to memory, through colonisation or family trauma, they come back to us through dreams and visions and visitations. So, there is a generic but also a rather specific nature of this learning. The totemic powers that guide and teach, guard and protect, that came from Elders teachings around the sacred fire, and that came to be associated with family and Two Spirit medicine practice. From our experience, these grew in awareness over many years. Others are different, and they come to know different energies. Native ways are flexible and must be personally relevant to you. Find your own path. Let this case be an example that may help you on that path of self-discovery. Learn your own story, as this is really the objective of learning. In our experience, the totemic Doors are Turtle in the north; Eagle in the east; Bear in the west; Wolf in the south.

Migjigi Turtle Nation

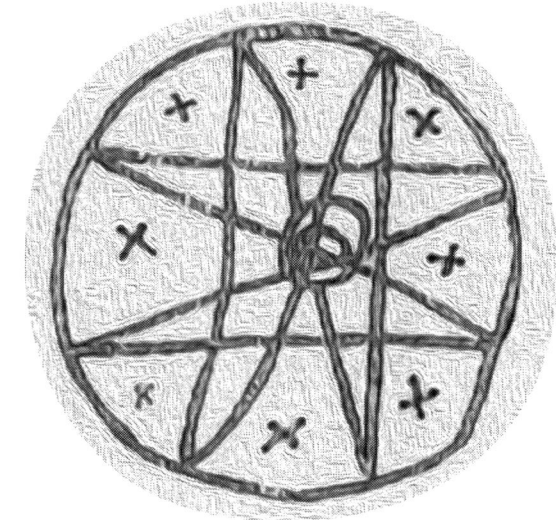

Muin Bear Nation   **Kitpu Eagle Nation**

Paq'tism Wolf Nation

The wisdom behind these Two Spirit teachings comes through the fact that Turtle is ancient Women's Medicine. We do not have time or space here to explore the depth of this teaching but let me simply say that there are so many wonderful layers and parts of this story that need to be appreciated and celebrated by Two Spirit people. Healing and birthing, and one of the oldest and formative first medicines of the planet.

Eagle medicine in the eastern door is also profoundly powerful and important to the Mi'kmaq nation. There are noble parts of Two Spirit medicine that require us to step up to national service. The foremost is that we carry the prayer of the nation by being in our bodies a Sacred Pipe. Eagle Pipe Medicine taught this teaching quite clearly. When carrying sacred medicine, we become that medicine. The reverse is also true, though more easily seen in retrospect.

Wolf medicine in the southern door is robust and powerful like the sun, giving life through the year, and playful and fierce in family ties and loyalty. Likewise Bear totem in the west guards the family and tribe and nation, giving strength through the long winter. To learn more about these teachings you may like to read my past book on the sacred teachings from the medicine lodge. You see in the cardinal totemic spirits a balance of forms and energies.

They are not gendered per se, but we might associate this. Turtle being Women's medicine. Wolf being Men's medicine. The poles of the wigwam spread out, but they join in sacred marriage of Turtle and Wolf. Eagle may be Men's medicine, and Bear Women's medicine. But different people will have their personal and familial ways. The connections respect and honour the women and men of Eskasoni, Bear River, Wildcat, and Waycobah and other communities who are always in prayers and visions. This too is a Two Spirit realisation. When you stand in the margins you don't go by formality and legality. You go by respect and loving acts of kindness Below you will see various associations. Again, this is only an example, as nothing in our traditions is dogmatic. Find your own way and live that way in beauty.

Mi'kmaq Wholistic Ecological Model

The model of ecology and life is wholistic. It works within the four directions of the compass. But these symbols represent a hologram, or web of associations. The model mirrors the complex systems sciences, and in fact incorporates ecological systems theory, life stage developmental theory, and a social-psychology steeped in notions of philosophical idealism, critical social theory, and phenomenology.

Sacred Direction: North

Life Stage: Elder

Sacred Moons: Kjiku's The Great Moon (December), Punamujuiku's Frost Fish Moon (January), Apiknajit Snow Blinder Moon (February)

Sacred Colour: White

Sacred Element: Water

Sacred Herb: Tobacco

Sacred Place: Spirit World

Sacred Helpers: Turtle, White Bear, Moose, Ant, Otter, Octopus

Life Passages: Emancipatory action; Integration & wisdom

Ecosystems: Metasystem (spirituality); Biosystem (planetary life)

Sacred Direction: East

Life Stage – Childhood

Sacred Moons: Siwkewiku's Spawning Moon (March), Penatemuiku's Egg Laying Moon (April), Etqoljewiku's Frog-croaking Moon (May)

Sacred Colour: Yellow

Sacred Element: Earth

Sacred Herb: Sweet Grass

Sacred Place: Earth World

Sacred Helpers: Bald Eagle, Deer, Mourning Dove, Lady Bug, Salmon

Life Passages: Discovery; Acknowledgement

Ecosystems: Microsystem (family); Mesosystem (community)

Sacred Direction: West

West – Life Stage: Adult

Sacred Moons: Wikumkewiku's Moose-calling Moon (September), Wikewiku's Animal-fattening Moon (October), Keptekewiku's River-freezing Moon (November)

Sacred Colour: Black

Sacred Element: Air

Sacred Herb: Sage

Sacred Places: World Beneath Water, World Beneath Earth

Sacred Helpers: Black Bear, Racoon, Buffalo, Squirrel, Worm, Trout

Life Passages: Critical reflection; Validation & resistance

Ecosystems: Chronosystem (socio-cultural history); Kairosystem (insight)

Sacred Direction: South

Sacred Moons: Nipniku's Summer Moon (Jun),

Peskewiku's Feather-shedding Moon (July), Kisikwekewiku's Fruit and Berry-Ripening Moon (Aug)

Sacred Colour: Red;

Sacred Element: Fire;

Sacred Herb: Cedar;

Sacred Places: World Above Earth, World Above Sky

Sacred Helpers: Wolf, Coyote, Dog, Golden Eagle, Snake, Spider, Dragon Fly, Whale

Life Passages: Affirmation; Disclosure

Ecosystems: Exosystem (political organisation); Macrosystem (culture and values)

Over many years we have developed these models and worked toward articulating an ecological and social science that supports healing, education, and post-colonial trauma-recovery. These models are worth exploring in as much as they convey pathways toward our future. The point here however is to share the Indigenous side of the story, and the wisdom and intuitive nature that creates the model. As much as possible however, we provide both sides of the brain-interface. For those readers who come from the Aboriginal cultural feeling and story-as-medicine, and for the western students of psychology and medicine who seek to understand 'how things work' piece by piece. To speak coherently to both ways of thinking is a delicate balancing act, and for most people this presents many challenges.

As the cognitive mind switches into concrete operational thinking, human beings tend to forget what life was like when thinking was actually more like feeling, sensing, and perceiving in a phenomenal world. This problem for people and the systems we have created is absolutely central to the local and global economic and environmental crisis we now face. It is also a key to unlock identity crisis, as people awaken from sleep. Life in this wholistic manner of perception holds its mystery, and synergies emerge more freely. Metaphors, dreams, stories, tales, lore, and the social nature of knowledge are more felt, embodied, because in the first instance knowledge is not actually or only cognitive. Knowledge in a pre-modern sense, even across all western cultures, was and remains primarily of the body and heart, and this is felt experientially, and this phenomenal experience registers as a wholistic, synergetic, and a complex systems-science-level-awareness. At the same time, Native thinkers are asked to 'rise up' into the phenomenal cognitive-mapping-two-eyed-seeing and perceive these many connections that already exist within our stories and tales. This bridge between worlds provides great and powerful medicine. In certain ways it takes a great deal of knowledge and skills in language to provide a truly holistic picture-in-words.

Several of our nation have told me the old ones used to keep their medicine pipes in the wigwam toward the top where they kept ledges or holders that hung from the beams of the tipi. This way the pipe was protected from being bumped plus it was bathed in the smoke of the wigwam and kept pure above the fire. This way the sacred pipe of the family was always ready to greet welcome to those who came to sit around the family fire. This image of the Two Spirit Old One of the People might be the best place to end this discussion for now... We wish you every peace on your path and wisdom in your heart and mind. May your family be protected and brought into light and peace for seven generations. May the Eagle rise in your sky, and Wolf stand behind your home in watchfulness. May the Bear keep you warm and strong during winters to come and may the Ancient Turtle Grandmother inspire your dreams and waking creations... Hold up the candle in the dark.

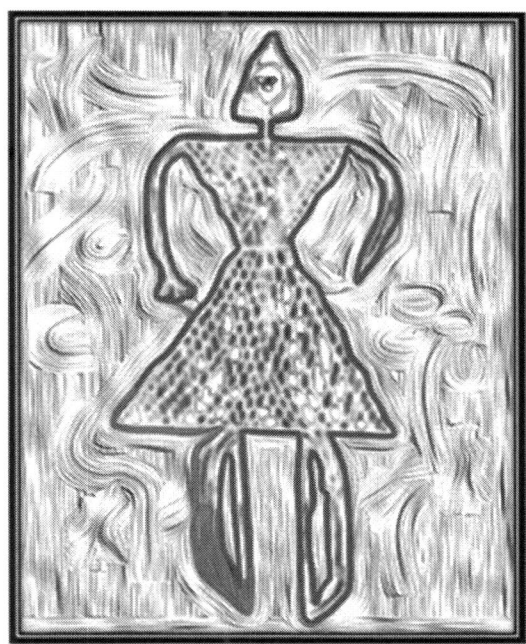

'Indigenous traditions teach about the importance of right perception and holding sacred the ordinary events and happenings of each day. By acknowledging the sacred we have built into our way of life a system of values and beliefs that honour the environment around us.'

Puoinaq Cultural Reawakening

Pjila'si, welcome, come in, sit down. Welcome to our sacred fire.

Debates over the nature of Mi'kmaw history and identity are can sometimes be extremely contentious. First Nation discourse has always been highly contested precisely because of its emergence within science, anthropology, and sociology. Aboriginal people were subjects for study. Now we refuse to be studied by others and have set up ethical and moral guidelines for research.

The current era is associated with Native self-government. This ideal is associated with defining the terms of our engagement with outside bodies. We seek to continue the dialogue but on a more equal footing. In relation to most areas of scholarship, until Native people take hold of the discourse and move forward on many levels, Aboriginal scholarship has slowed somewhat.

But more important in my mind is the cultural ground swell happening across Mi'kma'ki that is encouraging a cultural revival. Contrasting this are the opinions of certain Native academics who are critical of cultural reconstruction. My opinion is that culture is always undergoing evolution and change. Traditions are always being re-interpreted in each new generation. History does not stand still for anyone.

First Nation discourse tends to be unique in that we exist under an idealistic assumption based in 20th century humanism that we ought to live up to Mi'kmaw historical notions. In many ways people today are re-generating this myth. We are guilty of this in as much as we honour the pathways of Traditional Dreaming and Medicine Practice. But equally difficult is the tendency to throw out the baby with the bathwater, leaving behind anything that might spark the flames of stereotypes of the wise Indian elder, the mystic Indian, or the Medicine Woman. Many of our elders refuse to let go of Mi'kmaw spirituality and cultural identity.

What I appreciate most about cultural reconstruction is that this natural historical process lies quite outside of the hands of people like me and other scholars, professionals and intellectuals. We are not the people who move the ground swell. We are merely the ones who write commentary on an emerging cultural identity. And we should be more truthful, humble, and real about this fact.

Visions of Mi'kmaw Research-as-Ceremony

My work is about reflecting on cultural and spiritual identity. My focus is people today. I am not an historian, although I could write a fairly robust track on the historiography of Mi'kmaw ethnography over the years. In so saying, I am fairly critical of the work undertaken so far because existing writings do not reflect Mi'kmaw perspectives while clearly conveying historical biases and assumptions on the nature of Mi'kmaw culture from Euro-centric perspectives.

Please understand that I respect and deeply admire the foundational work of people like Ruth Holmes Whitehead. Ruth and I have known each other for several years. Her work has sincerely recovered much of Mi'kmaw stories, history and identity for current and future generations. However, she and I tend to agree that a new generation of research needs to be undertaken from a uniquely Mi'kmaw point of view.

This task ahead includes the area of gender and sexuality identity research that needs to be conducted by Mi'kmaw individuals who identify as Two Spirit, gay, lesbian, bisexual, transgender and/or intersex. The reason why this is necessary is because other researchers cannot gain the same level of awareness and sensitivity to the issues involved in being a minority within a minority within a minority.

Research into sexuality and gender variance shows that people without experience, awareness and training in these types of areas do not pick up the subtle cultural and hidden communications involved in minority contexts. When discussing this issue with Ruth while writing this chapter, she completely agreed that while she has been open minded about issues of gender variance and what she calls people of 'Two Natures,' she has not read the historical narratives from a mind-set of being trained and educated within and by the fields of gay and lesbian scholarship. She agreed with my estimation that it would require training of a Mi'kmaw researcher over several years, while perhaps supporting them through gaining a masters and perhaps also a doctoral program, to be adequately equipped to research these areas.

On one hand we need people who are well prepared to re-read the historical accounts, narratives and documents to look for cues, signs, and references to all the areas associated with gender variance, sexuality identity difference, and Two Spirit phenomena. On the other hand, we very much need people who are focused on gathering insider accounts of present day cultural and familial stories, memories and oral traditions associated with the topics at hand.

My work focuses on contemporary culture and how people make their sense of meaning. Within this, as part of my everyday life among Mi'kmaq friends and family I have gathered up perceptions gained from the oral tradition. But my focus has not been on actually gathering oral tradition stories as such. In this way, unlike Ruth I am not an ethnographer. My work is primarily focused within counselling psychotherapy, with a rather pragmatic view to offering people ways forward with strategies to assist with emotional, psychological and social issues of concern. In this sense, I am a healer and teacher.

Challenges Ahead

These are all pieces of work that are dearly needed, and I am hopeful that the Mi'kmaq Two Spirit community may be gathering their resources and focus to move some of these projects forward. It is therefore very important to state a number of issues clearly.

On one hand, there are currently no written historical references that I am aware of that suggest the historical Mi'kmaq had a Two Spirit tradition. Unlike tribes to the west where such references appear in the writings of Jesuit priests or other missionaries, or in other historical documentation, the likes of Ruth Holmes Whitehead tell me that such references have not yet been found in the Mi'kmaw historical record.

While I completely respect and trust Ruth's estimation on the written historical record, she and I mutually agree that in spite of her assessment there is the same need stated above for a new generation of minority researchers who can re-examine the historical narratives once trained in the sensitive nature of these issues. Elder Dr Daniel Paul's assessment confirms these insights. When you read his Foreword to this book you see a well thought out consideration of the historical nature of these issues. It is my opinion that until this study is adequately addressed by Two Spirit, gay or lesbian scholars we cannot confirm nor refute Ruth's determination on the written historical record.

In regard to the oral tradition, we must affirm that oral accounts hold incredible merit and weight within Indigenous research, both within the mainstream professions and from an Aboriginal cultural stance. The jury is not yet sitting to plan the gathering of data, let alone to determine some explanation of what the oral tradition has to say on the issue of Two Spirit identity and culture.

As far as I can tell so far, this work stands alone in this regard by gathering together this humble medicine bundle of a book. Likewise, from an historic view my career and research over many years may one day be seen as reflecting a Two Spirit focus. If so, so be it.

Mi'kmaw Oral Tradition

Suffice it to say that the oral tradition has much to tell us about Two Spirit Mi'kmaq phenomena. There are several important associations in the language that hold important clues to the nature of gendered ethics and sexuality identity among the Mi'kmaq Nation. Again, much emphasis appears to be placed on certain individual's roles to define the meaning of language, because so few people remain who have high levels of expertise in these areas.

There is a need for the sharing and rediscovery of insights among the Two Spirit Mi'kmaq. And we need to be free to engage in cultural reconstruction, if not to redefine historical identity, at least to set a clear path for Two Spirit youth.

While Ruth Holmes Whitehead expressed to me a rather clear and strong opinion on gendered identity that might exclude the possibility of a tradition associated with gender variance within her reading of the history, the stories and comments gained during my discussions with elders and members of the community suggest otherwise. In my analysis Ruth may be mistaken particularly given her timeframe for research was largely in decades past and during an era when these issues of gender and sexuality were far less talked about.

There seems to be a more fluid and perhaps largely hidden narrative that has truthfully been so taboo that it has never been spoken except in the quiet assurance of people like myself who are wholly non-threatening and whose identity poses no questions of being judged or evaluated. Ruth while so highly respected also carries authority in her work and person, an authority and respect as a woman, and as a person of European heritage. She is not

Two Spirit, and as such would not encourage these teachings and stories to come forward. It is not surprising that her research found no clues to this part of our cultural heritage.

It may also simply be that no one has asked the question before in such a clumsy and innocent manner as we might tend to do. Once people are over their initial shock and dismay, they seem to warm to the idea and quite enjoy a robust talk about what it is like being Two Spirited. Who they have known in their family. What was the Two Spirit role in history? How did they relate to women's medicine traditions, to men's medicine traditions?

It is also important to note how statistically unlikely the eventuality that there are absolutely no historical and cultural associations with gender variance among the Mi'kmaq, even if the written historical record proves to show no actual accounts or suggestions of the same. We ought to remember that according to all the best wisdom available to modern science people are inherently gender variant, prone to bi-sexuality both statistically and constitutionally, and every human society demonstrates same-gender preferences at one time or other.

We also must recall how historiography strongly suggests that histories need to be re-evaluated and rewritten from fresh perspectives, especially when dealing with colonial encounters. I am reminded of how many changes of perspective Elder Dr Daniel Paul's work has made to Mi'kmaq-European relations. His uncovering of historical records has thrown a completely different view of what had been a rather bland and misleading Euro-centric account. And yet, as we have suggested already, a gendered analysis of the historical record will most certainly reveal new insights.

In my study of gender variance and human sexuality over the past twenty-five years, I am convinced that there are occurrences of gender variant phenomena among every human society around the world. It is called many different names. Given divergent meanings and associations. Engenders different attitudes, beliefs and values. And manifests in many different forms of lifestyle and behaviour.

Science has concluded that as a species, human beings demonstrate the capacity to foster individuals whose gender and sexuality identity varies from the norm. Same gender love and intimacy is common among human beings. All the collective research into human sexuality, including hundreds and thousands of studies conducted by the Kinsey Institute in the USA suggest that human beings are in fact predominantly bisexual in nature. The human species has the capacity to love one another regardless of physical, gendered or sexual differences.

For these reasons, and as a psychotherapist, health sociologist, and sexologist I am convinced that there could be a strong case for the existence of an historical Mi'kmaq gender variant if not a Two Spirit tradition on more than one front. However, the hard work of drawing conclusions cannot be done until further research-as-ceremony is conducted.

The rest of this book will explore the meaning of Two Spirit as it is currently understood in the contemporary cultural context. While the debate over history may remain from the academic perspective the reality on the ground and in communities is plain sight acknowledgement of the Two Spirit path as both tradition and present-day practice. As a health and wellness practitioner this has in fact always been my primary area of work, to support people in what they believe and know today.

Body-based Memory

This is a contemporary story. This is about how people today see themselves and are making sense of their lives. Our story is our medicine. Our story is about how we experience our culture and spiritual ways. Our story is how we feel and think about our heritage. Within all of this, we deeply respect.

The phrase 'Two Spirit' comes from the North American Native traditions. As a pan-Indian phrase, the term relates to many traditions across Turtle Island. There is a story of its specific origin and there are widely felt links to its meaning within each nation. We seek to honour our Mi'kmaw ways.

This is a self-defining term among those of us who identify as Two Spirit in respect for our Native tradition. There is a growing appreciation and acknowledgement among many Native communities that speaks about acceptance and embracing of the Two Spirit way. This circumstance relates to the colonial history and how Christianity changed our communities and our ways of being. But also, how we seek a deeper healing and recovery of our ways.

The Two Spirit way teaches us about who we are. We all carry laws in our bodies, minds, hearts, and spirits that are also on-going regardless whether we are aware or remain blind. These laws govern our lives in ways we cannot escape. We ignore these basic laws to our own demise. When we fall off the path we mess things up. When we live in balance and beauty, life blossoms and resilience grow.

These ancient and ecological laws are in-tune within the environment, the ecology of the Earth World. These sacred teachings exist across the Six Worlds. These laws are expressed in the Medicine teachings. These laws come forward in the Sacred Fire, Sweat Lodge, Vision Quest, Sunrise Ceremony, and in many other Ceremonies of the First Peoples. In this moment it is not for me to explain these laws. It is only necessary to suggest that each person needs to learn these ways. How do we learn? By leaning into the fire and watching the coals. As your awareness shifts, move from the fire to the heart. Listen more deeply. This is how we learn the sacred ways. In this natural and personal way, what is real now for you comes alive. This is how your way of listening makes your culture a part of who you are.

When it comes to sexuality and spirituality, we carry the 'blueprint' of these laws in our body. Certain persons remember and can articulate these Medicine Teachings. We often call these Medicine Keepers. We don't say Medicine Makers. We say Keepers. The sacred laws already exist, we do not make them up. Medicine people listen and learn. They awaken to the ways. Then at some stage they teach to others who are also listening.

The Medicine Keepers are the same as anyone else. Yes. They only listen longer and more closely. They sit with the Medicines many years. They do this to listen and to learn. Any person can walk this path, though few people choose to devote so much time and silence to learning and to listening.

This means people who keep Medicine are often humble and servants of the community. They know the more you learn and listen, the more there is to learn. The quieter you become. The more you realise you know very little. Life is one great big mystery. And the path is endless.

You will know a Medicine Person by how they put their own identity to the side, how they focus on the teachings. For them, the Medicine is the focus. The Way of the Pipe is the silent guide for their work. First and foremost, the Two Spirit way is a Medicine way.

What do we hear when we listen to the Two Spirit Medicine? First, we hear love. Two means not just one. Two means energy coming together. Two is community. Two is bonding in listening, communicating, and loving. Sit with this silence long enough and you will hear the Old Medicine like an Ancient Dance, a Sensual Two-Legged Music, like the roots of two trees conjoining under the fragrant earth.

The human spirit seeks freedom to love. You have man. You have woman. They are destined to come together. They seek each other out, and begin to communicate, listen, and love. The ceremony of their lives creates family. Children are born from this joining of one and one. From solitary nature comes two. Two in love make a new oneness. So, each and every child is sacred. Over eons man and women grow and interweave their magic and forms. Individual medicine paths cross over.

In this cross over a Two Spirit being is born. This is happening in the Spirit World and then in the World of Our Ancestors. The being crosses over into the Two Spirit ways, they then spend time with our Ancestors in the World of the Stars. They trace across the expanse of the universe. They chase the Great Bear in flight. They learn from the Old Ones of the People. In that place they sit by the sacred fire of the elders. Many eons pass. Worlds come and go. Then in a twinkle of an eye a Two Spirit is born into this skin-time.

A youthful Two Spirit is already ancient. Yet they are born into skin-time once again. A new baby Two Spirit. They have very much to learn. The transformation is a migration from one solitary spirit to being of the Two Spirit way. Like a Loon travels to another country from far south into the lakes of Mi'kma'ki to raise their young. They must let go and take nothing with them on this journey. In the same way we leave behind the male spirit and female spirit and take on a new Two Spirit way. In this the Two Spirit being takes on new power. New medicine. New teachings. None of this happens in any visible way. We cannot prove this teaching. We only observe this in our children born into our families. We can only listen and learn. We can only listen and learn by living this story, remembering this deep abiding truth. You will know if this is true just by listening and learning.

Two-legged want to love without restrictions. To do this, human beings must follow their heart. Following the heart in the ancient ways honours ethics of care, compassion, service, humility, and justice. But like St Augustine once said, 'Love and do what you want.' The ethics of love is limitless. Creation itself is a garden that we native people never had to leave. We did not sin and were not cast out. Our innocence remains. At the core of this innocence is our medicine ways. The centre of the medicine ways is the sacred fire. In the flames and coals of that fire are the Two Spirit beings of power. They are Kisiku Sa'qewei Kji Puoinaq – Ancient Elder Two Sprit with Great Power.

In contrast and hard to say when speaking this sacred mystery, we listen and learn that in the European and American lineage there are many value conflicts, wars, and disease that place two legged in harm's way. Disconnection from Mother Earth leads to conflict that dishonours the Original Instructions of the Ancestors of all tribes of humanity. These one-sided politics support forms of power that diminish humanity. The cult of the individual is extreme. Two legged try to right the wrongs and imbalance of the past in reactionary cycles of trans-generational trauma. Coming back to the original wisdom is difficult for many, though not impossible.

We native people need our own way. We need our own grounding and balance in our Medicine traditions. The Two Spirit way is one of these Sacred traditions that the Seventh Generation is awakening for the sake of our People.

Some say that Aboriginal people rely on a collective consciousness to the exclusion of individual thought. This is misleading. Old Medicine ways in most Indigenous Nations press the importance of gaining personal skills, awareness, and discernment. The individual stands strong within their traditions. A warrior knows who they are by standing strong within the family, tribe, and nation.

A strong nation depends on strong spirits-in-flesh to carry the teachings forward. Each of us are the Ancestors for the seventh generation who are coming down the line. So, we carry this awareness of our personal and community responsibility. In these ways the person is in balance with family, tribe, and nation. Not one single thing is more important than all the rest. All are of equal importance and sacredness. Even so, many of us when in right-mind and heart would give our lives for the family, tribe, and nation. Our love is complete.

Decolonising the Sacred Sexual

Euro-American systems of governance are based on a false premise. They make one small insight a universal and absolute truth. For example, they say that the church is all important. They say the government or king is to be obeyed at all costs. They say today that the rights of the individual outweigh the rights of the community. These extremes are false and illogical.

In contrast, Aboriginal frameworks are logical and balanced. The Native Red Road is a wholistic framework for working out difficult and complex problems that face humanity. This form of logic is wholistic – so it also involves listening to vision, intuition, many and varied perspectives. These processes of gaining balanced answers to the issues facing humanity demand much integrity and selflessness. One simple answer is unfeasible. Making a simple answer universal and absolute is dangerous to our survival. We have to do the hard work of staying with the problems long enough to find wholistic solutions. Listen and learn. Listen and learn.

This is important when we want to understand the Two Spirit way. We need to let go of the ideas the mainstream has fed to us about human sexuality. The mainstream's own ideas about human sexuality are based on a sad history of psychopathology.

Not many people realise that the word 'heterosexual' was created after the word 'homosexual' to contrast against what was looked at as deviant and sinful. Thus, the whole idea of human sexuality that evolved since the late 19th century was hindered by Christian hell fire and shame-based beliefs that remain to this day. The word homosexual came first, and heterosexual followed, arising from sexology studies on incarcerated men, and were created in the last two decades of the 19th century. They did not exist prior to this time. How they ended up in the Christian Bible and were considered valid translations is a story that is entirely absurd. How Christians today claim to hate the homosexual 'sin' but to love the 'sinner' is equally difficult to understand.

More to the point, to understand the actual social intersections between colonial imperialist Christian social beliefs and practices and Mi'kmaw cultural and cosmological approaches that waxed and waned during the colonial encounter over the past several hundred years, we need what Elders Albert Marshall calls two eyed seeing. In this case, two eyed seeing must stretch into a form of historiography, sociology, and critical social theory that are based within an Indigenous standpoint approach to analysis and critique.

For example, we can examine the social histories and values around terms like E'pit, Epitejijewe'k, Puoinaq, Kistele'k, and misunderstood/misused terms like Geenumu Gessalagee which also have their unique histories, and points of insight and/or wisdom to reveal. We can examine colonial and dominant concepts like baptism and their social and liturgical practices over time, and map changes in beliefs and practices like gendered social norms that can be traced in historical accounts and understood through the ways these social norms change at certain periods of history. We can then realistically construct a map of the parallel processes that may be occurring in Mi'kmaw history even while the details have not been documented. By tracing social ideas and practices like this, we can come to a better understanding of notions of gender, social life, family life, as well as spirituality, beliefs, and the interactions between cosmologies and religious/cultural practices.

This book is but the first step in this process of sociological and historical deconstruction and reconsideration. So are Elder Dr Paul's historical works. Elder Professor Marie Battiste's work is also part of this first generation of reconstructive scholarship. But more important perhaps, these efforts are socially, culturally, and spiritually grounded within a community and a national context and represent medicine pathways that hold a great deal of significance for the healing of many nations.

By taking these insights further, how might we view the colonial social values including the Christian mentalities of the 17th, 18th, 19th, and 20th centuries, respectively? It is important to realise that these beliefs and practices were by no means consistent! This begs the question of how can things change so much, and remain so much the same? To answer this, we must first realise that things change for the oppressor all the time. But beyond being put in their place and forced to comply, things rarely change for the oppressed. Using the principles of a pedagogy of the oppressed that was first articulated in modern times within the Latin American context (Freire, 1978) we can apply two eyed seeing practices of analysis to a backward gaze upon the colonial encounter and examine the dual layers of colonial discourse in relation to minority oppression. As it were, during each phase of history over the past 500 or more years. We say 'or more' because no historical reflection is adequate unless it includes analysis of the times, contexts, and conceptual origins influencing those times under study.

The importance of this analysis for future studies comes to light lately as we examine the social fabric of concepts that contribute to Two Spirit reflections. For example, Mi'kmaw cultural ways suggest that people are whole beings and need to be respected for their inherent integrity. We do not separate conduct from personhood. We know what you do is who you are, period. We call this honour and integrity. We call this respect. The historical colonial and Christian sense of integrity shifted and changed during the centuries. Just looking at the Victorian era we can track significant change in notions of honesty, propriety, gender relations, keeping face, defence of honour, etc… It is simply not possible to say that conduct and personhood were fused in the same way that was common in Mi'kmaw culture. For the Victorian it was absurd and simplistic to attach what a person does to who that person is in character and value. In fact, action was in many ways entirely independent from the value of a person. The latter may be based in a range of factors, including social standing, family affiliation, nobility, social role, wealth, or profession.

At the same time, we cannot over simplify Mi'kmaw cultural values. However, accounting for variance and contextual factors within the life of an oppressed people, it stands to reason that the colonial culture and its Christian variants had and continue to have different sets of values. The difference can be studied, and understood in greater detail, leading toward a better understanding of the range of factors important to Mi'kmaw and Two Spirit emancipation.

When you analyse power in society it is helpful to ask, who is gaining the most? Who is gaining social power by imposing this belief, value, or law? Who stands to benefit and how?

Traditionally native ways do not impose or enforce. Native ways invite and discuss, welcome and embrace. We build by consensus. If a native person disagrees they can walk away. Native autonomy is sacred, because every being is sacred. Consensus includes other non-two-legged creatures. All of these concepts, beliefs, and practices are radically different from the colonial cultural status quo. In this creation-based approach of the Mi'kmaq there is nothing extra needed to make a good person. We are already good in our being. All creation is good. This is why Two Spirit and LGBTIQ+ people are at basis accepted by many within the traditional cultural values. We say 'at basis' because of course acceptance is awesome, but equally, people show their true colours as they live, act, and do whatever they do in life. A person's value to the family, tribe, and nation is also part of this capacity to measure a person based on their inherent ability to walk the red road, so to speak. For example, to be kind, loving, forgiving, patient, giving, and of service to others.

All of us along with our Two Spirit family members can gain so much by rediscovering and reclaiming our Sacredness. Our sacred nature challenges many of the dominant ways of knowing in the worlds of today. Our sacred sexuality challenges both mainstream and Indigenous contexts as we heal from colonial values.

In the same way in our native cultures two legged beings may be this way and that way, but they have never really been 'male' and 'female' in the sense defined by European-Canadian cultures. In Mi'kmaw ways, a person was often defined more by what they were good at doing. A person who loved to weave became known as a weaver. Another who loved to fish, and hunt took on these roles and qualities, gifts and talents. Anyone of any gender might do these things. The sex of the person was secondary, hardly worth mention. What that person contributed to family and nation was the focus, and how they loved others was the point of honour.

Because perceptions of the Two Spirit path have diverged away from family and tribal life since the invasion of foreign values and beliefs, today we are recovering these connections. We are perhaps learning and listening more deeply to these tides that have been present but hidden in plain view.

Part of our pathwork relies on resetting our being within ancient cosmology. The cosmology of our nation is profound. Incredible. Worth many years of sitting, listening, and learning. Cosmology is how we map our worlds and make sense of life. Cosmology is how we sense the universe fits together into a meaningful circle, or more like it, a cycle of circles and spirals that dance and weave a very grand mystery. Reconstructing both Two Spirit and Mi'kmaq culture wait upon the new generations to live within these wholistic and integral ways.

Mi'kmaw Cosmology

Essentially, everything in Mi'kmaq traditional language and culture appears sacred. There is a whole and complete sacred world woven together by Kisu'lk, the One Who Made Everything. We call Kisu'lk the Great Spirit, Kji Niskam. These words do not suggest gender.

In the traditional way it is not important whether the Creator Spirit is male or female. Elders say forms of the ancient words for Creator conveyed non-gender, both genders, and either/or genders all at the same time. This notion of the Creator is very important. In fact, the quality of shape shifting is hidden in this meaning. Creator is dynamic. You cannot pin down a great mystery. Two legged beings are the same, although we forget this because we think we are all just ordinary. How sad and pathetic when we are just so ordinary. But when you realise we are made of star dust and divine power, you begin to catch the deeper meanings in native language. Native language remembers the great mystery and wonders of the universe.

As we are saying gender is not central to Mi'kmaw spirituality. Mi'kmaw theology and cosmology are creation-focused and did not begin with a man and women as father and mother of all peoples. The creation stories suggest diversity in creation, and great mystery, and the roles of beings like Gluscap who helped Creator to form the land and sea. There are families in creation stories, not simply male and female. There are a people who emerge from the mystery of Mother Earth.

In Mi'kmaw ways, Creator is unique, set apart as sacred yet part of everything all at once. My heart appreciates this approach because the Energy of Evolution, of Creation, is found within all things. And all things are not bound by gendered definitions as tends to happen in many European traditions and languages.

Mi'kmaw cosmology and spiritual ways honours Naku'set, the Sun. The Sun travels in a circle and gives its energy because of being created by Kji Niskam. The Sun gives us the day to produce and work, to co-create with Kji Niskam. The Sun is gracious and grants us the peace of night to rest. Giver of light, heat and warmth the Sun provides the energy for plants and animals to grow and have life.

Naku'set is full of Power and Sacred Clarity. In my experience, the Mi'kmaq People respect Naku'set very much. At times I have stood with Elders around the Sacred Fire, listening to the sounds of the Sacred Drum and the Ceremonial Leader chanting in traditional language. Early before dawn, in the still quiet of the last watch of night. During the clear skies when the Milky Way can be seen across the expanse of the World Above the Sky. Waiting in anticipation and reverence for the Rising of the Dawn. Naku'set first appears by rays of light that change the nature of the cosmos in subtle shades, and the anticipation grows... As rational as I may be, when Naku'set arrives and peaks first above the horizon my heart is filled with an intensive warmth and contentment. We are People of the Dawn.

We live in the Earth World, Wsitqamu'k. This is uniquely the Mi'kmaq People's World, where we walk, make love, share in the life of all creatures, and enjoy the fruits and berries of this land. Naku'set was given the task to watch over the Sacred Land and all of her peoples. In this way, we live in a cosmology that generates a feeling of relationship, family and kinship. In this kind of world everything is Sacred, and nothing is hidden from view.

When you listen to the stories, Kluskap was created after Wsitqamu'k was formed by Creator, and after the plants, animals and birds were placed on the surface of the earth. Creator formed Kluskap with a bolt of lightning that hit Wsitqamu'k and created the form of an image of a human body. His body was formed from the first element of the land, sand. Another bolt of lightning gave life to Kluskap. But he was still held fast by the earth and was unable to move. He lay there and watched Naku'set travel across the Sky World. His head lay in the direction of the rising sun. His feet were in the west. His arms were stretched out towards north and south. For a long time, he lay there. He watched the world come and go around him, the animals and plants grow and live and die. He asked Kisu'lk to give him the ability to move about the Mi'kmaw world. It was then that a third crash of lightening came from Creator that allowed Kluskap to stand on the surface of the earth and to walk freely about the world.

His first action was to turn around in a circle seven times. He then looked up at the Sky World and gave thanks to Kisu'lk. He then looked down upon Wsitqamu'k and offered thanks for giving him the sand that made his body, and again gave thanks to Kisu'lk. He then looked inside himself and gave thanks to Kisu'lk for giving him soul and spirit. He then turned his attention to give thanks to the Four Directions and opened his heart to acknowledging the connections with all of the earth and the world around him.

Slowly over time Kluskap explores the phenomenal world of the Mi'kmaq Nation, and slowly one by one, his family comes to live with him. First his Grandmother. Then his nephew. Then his mother. Over time he learns the basic lessons of life and how to live well and true. Toward the end of life in the Mi'kmaw world he and his family leave important teachings to the People including to honour the Sacred Fire from which he was first formed.

From the original stories passed down there is a sense of the importance of learning, listening, watching and coming to know the world around us. These patterns of behaviour are taught and experienced by the People. Women and men exist in the world, but their existence is a spiritual and phenomenal experience. Women are held as Sacred not because they are female, but because they are the portals through which all spirits enter the Mi'kmaw Earth World to learn the lessons they are meant to learn.

Women are the First Medicine. This is not a gender specific role in the western sense. This is a spiritual purpose and destiny. Men are meant to serve and support women in their caring and nurturing roles. But can I say that gender is not mentioned or acknowledged in any overt sense of the terms. People are rather viewed as spiritual entities given flesh and bones to carry them around. In fact, human beings as spiritual entities can change shape, shape-shift, and can manifest different spirits. These stories of shape-shifters and of how they too go about the worlds learning various lessons are also part of the cosmology of the Mi'kmaq people.

In my exposure to Mi'kmaw teachings and stories, I am given to feel a deep philosophy of embodiment and of spiritual independence from embodiment are aspects of the largely unspoken nature of culture. Kluskap's way of being formed by Creator suggests complete dependence on the spiritual power of lightening to first generate form, then substance, and then movement. There are the physical, the spiritual, and the temporal aspects of existence. Each has its own depth and wonder. The ways that Kluskap went about his phenomenal world suggest a child learning what it means to be alive, and to be in relationship with the world around us. These are great mysteries to be discovered. There is much wisdom to gain and then to be shared. A cultural template for learning and for social relations is set down within these and other old stories. And they are quite wonderful and essential parts of cultural learning.

Kluskap like all Mi'kmaq have a purpose in the world of being in relationship with their Grandmother, Nephews, Nieces, Mothers and all other members of the family. The identity of the man is about maintaining respectful relations and supporting family members. These ways of respect are essential to survival in the tribe. In my estimation, Kluskap did not choose to be male. Creator made him a being of power.

The Elders who created and sustained these ancient stories gave us many clues and hints as to the nature of human spiritual identity. Today we might apply this awareness to our contemporary notions. But we need to take care, because we should not impose a western gendered idea onto the Mi'kmaw tradition. People today in our communities are highly influenced by these gendered norms. And they are extremely difficult to put aside.

The Kluskap cycle gives much food for thought. Kluskap is not necessarily a male who finds a female and has children. His role in life is quite unique. He is born in three stages, and yet he is fully formed as a man once he is freed from the earth. In ways he seems to be set apart like a holy man or Medicine Man. In native traditions this type of Spirit Being is often a Two Spirit. A being who is male-bodied or female-bodied and yet walks through the world in a spiritual manner that connects with the energy and purpose of women and men. In many respects we can see this quality and dynamic in the Kluskap cycle.

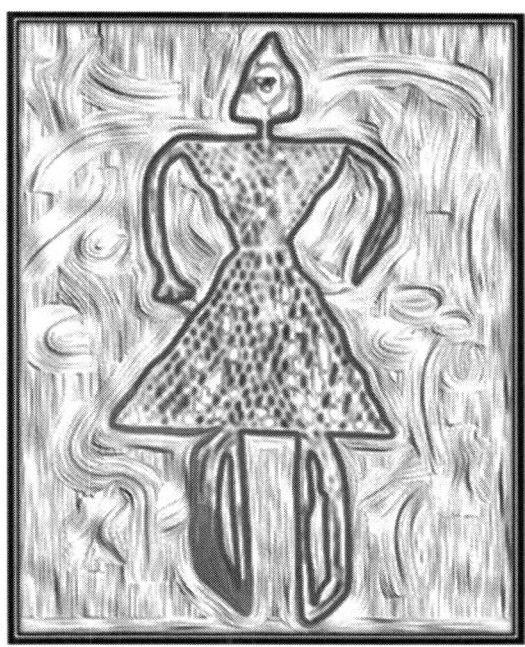

'Colonial histories have led to great imbalances of ethical and moral values that have eroded people's relationships with local, regional and national ecosystems. Loss of what we might consider traditional Indigenous cultural values has allowed communities and societies to dominate and abuse the land and exploit its natural resources… Threats to cultural diversity combine with ecological harm, resulting in less access to important knowledge and wisdom – leaving all human beings more vulnerable.'

Two Spirit Medicine Teachings

Pjila'si, welcome, come in, sit down. Welcome today on this historic day to our sacred fire. Why today? Because you have come this far, and you are still here, listening… Come closer, stay warm.

Two Spirit Medicine is a study of the cultural and spiritual meaning and purpose of those members of the native community who are in certain ways set apart and acknowledged as having medicine. Traditional medicine is many things. In a sensory-experiential and integral philosophy of life, medicine is wholistic. Health is based in wholism, not so much its parts, but how parts of health fit together and co-create balance, equipoise, stasis, and change. This ecological model of integral studies and two eyed seeing incorporates a broad spiritual and value-based quality of being. When abiding with maleness, femaleness, two-spirit-ness, we see these qualities, dimensions, and fields of being including what today are material layers of gender variance, sexuality, sexual practice, and sexual health. But now you can understand more readily how these latter parts are only a part of the whole. As such, you can also see the inappropriate ways that sexual health as a field imposes upon the Mi'kmaq and other Indigenous nations.

We can also understand that the capacity to love members of their own gender is only a very small and a rather unimportant part of how Indigenous culture values a person overall. Who we sleep with is less important than who we are in the eyes of our Elders. And this is kind of what really counts. This is also what calls us younger ones to maturity, integrity, and honour. This is how values are manifest more likely through the gifts and talents we display. In some circumstances, Two Spirit people are set apart not so much because of any mundane gender or sexual variance, but more so because they have attained a high degree of cultural, familial, tribal or spiritual knowledge and skill.

A highly respected Two Spirit within Mi'kmaw culture is more likely to be a person of high standing because of their hard work, commitments, and longstanding integrity and personal wisdom than for any other reason. That they are Two Spirit means little unless this part of their person is integrated into their makeup such that this deepens and opens their perceptions and abilities. For example, a person may be identified as gay or lesbian. They may identify this way themselves. They may not be seen or identify personally as Two Spirit because they have not gone down that road and have not become that person yet. They may have a long-time partner of the same gender and simply identify as gay, because that is the most practical label they have at the moment.

The more hidden processes involved in this transformation of self toward the Two Spirit identity may be an aspiration. It may take many years to grow into this being. We have explored the processes of growth and healing of self and family involved in Two Spirit awakening. We can understand from this therapeutic perspective how the Elder's teachings around healing of the nation are often linked into the recovery of the Two Spirit ways. Like most spiritual and ecological paths, the development of the human being involves our families and nation. When one being awakens, many if not all beings become a bit lighter. Those closer by tend to be affected the most.

Certainly, part of this awakening is shifts in personal values, beliefs, attitudes, and the sense of awakening to the possibility of being something more. Other aspects of this involve ceremonial initiation into the Power of Spirit. This holds a fascination for me. Ceremony from my view is therapeutic and educational. Ceremony is based in lived experience. There is little academic or theoretical about ceremony and therapy that is well done. Good therapy gives people an actual experience of healing, of change of mind or heart. Experience allows a person to register in body the actual felt-sense of change. Ceremony is the same when done well, with good intentions.

Initiation Ceremonies

Initiation ceremonies tend to prepare people for life-passages. For example, the ceremonies of infants in arms with their mother prepare them for first attempts at crawling and walking. Positive attachment with parents gives infants the resilience and strength they need for the excitement and scary world of stepping away from their main source of safety and comfort.

In similar ways, initiation ceremonies during childhood and youth prepare a young person for entry into puberty when they take another step away from the secure attachments of parents and close family ties, and they venture into the worlds of dating, meeting strangers, and exploring the wider world. In older times we had initiation ceremonies proper, and many still practice forms of these ceremonies. A first hunt is one of the ways that boys and girls so inclined may take up adult roles and be initiated into forms of leadership and greater responsibility. Learning to crochet and do basket weaving can be important ceremonial moments for youth just as well. In the Mi'kmaw culture these practices are highly valued and shared by women and men.

In a society where our cultural roles have been confused by colonisation, gender roles related to initiation can also become a bit muddled. But people tend to sort through these issues by simply focusing on celebrating seasonal and annual events and gatherings and caring for each other within the family. So, at this everyday level there are ways that people celebrate and initiate into gifts and talents that may relate to either gender including becoming a parent. Clearly being a father and a mother are unique but sharing parenting is also largely the circle that culture shares. If we are serious about being parents taking a male quality or female quality tends to be flexible for people who understand this deeper cultural way. A mother takes on the roles of father, a father the roles of mother. Healthy relationships often go this way.

Two Spirit roles may overlap these gender roles, and/or take on a new and different quality when a person moves further along the initiatory path of Two Spirit Medicine. These teachings have largely been forgotten but will return to people when they are ready.

One pathway to this knowledge rests in the Elder's teachings that the Two Spirit being is a highly evolved soul who has lived many lifetimes in human form, and who has come to balance the spirits of male and female, such that they can carry the Sacred Medicine Bundles of both men and women's Dreaming. The Two Spirit being may also or alternatively embody two Powerful Spirits, such as that of the Kitpu and Paq'tism, the Eagle and the Wolf. Perhaps several other spirits embodied. To actually attain this standing in the spiritual realms is quite an accomplishment of the Creator that is signalled by a deeper sense of humanity, humility and service to others.

Penetrating wisdom pierces the heart and soul to such a great degree, like lightning struck our cultural hero Kluskap, and they were allowed by power and protection in Two Spirit Medicine to greet the stone faces who arrived in the large wooden canoes from the east. They were travelling the waters of the great lake. Medicine Keepers were travelling the intuitive waters of being. These waters link together where the gulf opens to the sea. In those waters fresh mixes with salt. In this manner we taste the ways that human agency transforms into spiritual power. This is the Two Spirit path. Found where the gates of the Eastern Door open out into the expansive waters of being.

If these suggestions hold any truth it actually means that the Two Spirit path contains many basic truths that can assist people on their journey to spiritual wholeness. While rooted in the cultures of native North America, these teachings have a much wider application and relevance. I am sure that a part of these mysteries rests with the fact that the Two Spirit person attains within their body a blending and integration of masculine and feminine powers, leading to a more whole and complete person. Indeed, Two Spirit is all of this and more than this. Human beings live gender as much as we transcend to a higher plane of existence. We love and become love. The spiritual energy of love includes and greatly transcends.

We Two Spirits see this nature of love in particular form and in transcendence by experience of our totemic powers. The ways that the spirits of our four legged, winged, finned, crawling, and leafy kin actually move within our lives. This teaches us by ways of initiation. Through spirit pathways we learn and grow.

On one hand we two legged are so disconnected. So alienated. Yet on the other hand we are deeply connected. We only need to breathe deeply. To accept. To open heart and mind. There is fear for some of us, for most of us. Yet we learn from fear like a brother and sister. Fear is a good teacher when we refuse to react and close down. When we listen, we can open our heart and mind to initiation into our totemic powers. We can walk with the wolf, the eagle, the otter… We can sing with the bear, the crow, the hummingbird. We can learn much by visits to the World Beneath the Earth or the Water World. We can take a path into the World Above the Sky. There are many ways to learn.

Two Spirit initiation provides experiential wisdom to open this dynamic ceremonial educaring world. Yes, there are parallels in men's medicine and women's medicine. And many Elders we have sat with share a deep abiding intuition that Two Spirit Medicine practices rest within that highly regarded space, in that Wigwam of Medicine Keepers, where some of the very wise Old Ones of the People have sat and continue to guide us. When we are ready to listen and learn. We may find ourselves within this chamber of ancients still sitting around the earthy fire of service and humility.

Men's and Women's Medicine

Within this we need to also acknowledge that for native and Aboriginal people around the world, men's business and women's business are temporal and spiritual domains of knowledge, skill, ability, capacity and wisdom-teachings that convey a profound wealth of human and spiritual awareness. For Indigenous people gender is not reduced to male and female body parts and sexual relations, end of story. Each Medicine holds many stories, teachings and methods of working in the world that open pathways to personal power, accomplishment, and growth towards spiritual enlightenment.

Having such incredible honour to sit and learn from Aboriginal Australian Elders, and from Canadian Indian Elders, there is a sense in my life now of the depth of richness of our Indigenous heritage. Our ways are many and one, given to local knowledge and opening up into the ocean of common values of respect and honour.

As the Kluskap legends suggest, we are given life in this phenomenal world to learn the lessons we are meant to learn. We are the Stars who Sing. We Sing with our Light. The essential and energetic nature of reality is central to Mi'kmaw cosmology. Our primary purpose is not to be male or female and to dominate the earth. Our primary purpose is to be, to learn, and then to offer our teachings to others and go back into the Spirit World. Our children are our Song Lines given in love. The spiritual nature of childhood teaches us as adults to rekindle the fires of learning, wonder, and respect for life. Our children are our medicine.

One of the more potent Two Spirit prophecies that has come to my awareness relates to the saying that when the Two Spirit are fully embraced things will change. The story goes that when the most despised and misunderstood members of native culture since the early days of colonization are accepted and held up as part of the heart of the nation – only then will the native people heal from their past trauma and move forward with power and strength. The saying is lovely simply for its childlike wisdom. Who can represent the wonder of creation more than a Two Spirit child or a Two Spirit of high degree whose actual life is dedicated to childlike wonder, learning, service, and respect. In another way of speaking, when the most vulnerable in society are held up as our medicine then the people will become strong again.

This rings true if you consider that colonisation has attacked the heart of the Mi'kmaq people's ethics which focus on the centrality of women, elders, and children. Men's role in the traditional sense is to care for these members of the nation because our future belongs to women and children, while our past belongs to the elders. This is a big circle. Our future actually belongs to our elders who sing for their seventh generation to come. This powerful truth comes home when visited by our elders from long ago, who share their story and prayers. We can simply remember. We have seen this in therapy and ceremony and through the experiences shared around the fire. In Aboriginal cultures time is a circle and is not so much a clean line from past to future or future to past. A person can be in many places at one time.

Time wise take note that Kluskap has around him his Grandmother, Mother, and Nephew. Two women elders and one youth. One elder, one parent, one child. The whole human lifespan. Also, the future, present, and past. The past, present, and future. All together with Kluskap two males and two females. Each with their own spiritual purpose. All four together forming a family. Four Doors – North, South, East, and West. But not in a gender binary. Rather there is diversity in creation. A Two Spirit Medicine keeper who happens to be male. A mother who happens to be female. A grandmother who happens to be female. A child who happens to be male. An emphasis on the feminine pathways including Two Spirit wisdom and power, which in the tradition tends to be highly regarded within the medicine of giving life and nurturing creation. Creation tends to be a feminine power. Serving this power is the masculine energy and youthful energy. The Mi'kmaw way is about balance of spiritual energies, the Four Sacred Directions, giving harmony to the sands that gave Kluskap life through the power of the lightning bolts. The cosmology balances our lives and sets us into our place of power, our purpose and sense of meaning. This is who we are, the L'nu, the People.

In a similar way, the Two Spirit sees in this story celestial harmony working itself out through creative agency, emerging tensions, familial relations, and harmonic resonance with spiritual entities and powers - All Our Relations. This is the Two Spirit Mi'kmaw Path. Creative and wonderful. Alive and dynamic. Giving life to the People.

Two Spirit Service and Skill

Where the Two Spirit comes into this picture is quite fascinating. Mi'kmaw Elders highly respected tell me that the traditional role of the male-bodied Two Spirit is to be a servant to women, elders, and children while other members of the society are focused on their active roles of hunting and gathering. Female-bodied Two Spirit often take on the roles of hunting with the other men, although these generalizations cannot contain the diversity of roles and talents that each person carries.

Several elders expressed to me that while men and women were separated during women's moon time, this was not due to a rigid separation of gender roles. This was due to the spiritual nature and power of women's moon time, during which they needed to take a step away from men. They may take time away to a sacred place of medicine and the younger women or others not on their moon time would manage the tasks of daily life. A grandmother may spend time with a young woman coming into her first moon times. Cultural and spiritual teachings surrounded these experiences.

What became the moon tide taboo was first associated with honour and respect for women's spiritual power as Givers of Life. This teaching still holds power among the L'nu. The moon tide flows like the Sacred Waters of the River. We are part of creation; how could this not be so? Entering into this flow of nature and giving this gift of life back to Mother Earth is spiritually for the renewal of the land, sea, and all the people.

Women's moon time being connected with the power of sacrifice, childbirth, and service to family and creation were and continue to be deeply respected. Integral to the cosmology and cultural ways of the L'nu. Part and parcel of the ways that Elder women, mothers, aunts, and sisters take on the roles of helping one another to prepare for and deal with the pressures and responsibilities of women's roles and medicine.

The metaphorical, mystical, and spiritual quality of human experience in women's medicine is also present in men's medicine. Men share places and times that are initiatory in nature such as during the hunt, sitting and talking, eating and having a drink of water during the hike or when in canoe on the lake. Stories and teachings are shared. Joke and fun around male body functions are normal parts of life in these spaces. The more serious teachings around male roles and perhaps also body functions would be discussed privately or in more general ways around the fire during these times when Elder men, fathers, and sons were together. Before and after significant ceremonies like Sweat men may traditionally share and discuss issues important to each person. A turning point like a first hunting or fishing trip, or first portage to another lake or region, may also be times of sharing. Preparing for taking on the roles of partner and father were also significant times for male Elders and fathers to invest in the care of their sons.

Often humility and deference for privacy guard the ways that body functions are discussed across both spaces for women and men. In the older ways of wisdom, teachings involve the spiritual purpose and nature of body functions. Both tend to speak to how we are water and life, and that giving our being for the creation is part of our purpose. Woven into the nature of our being two legged.

Two Spirit Purpose and Vocation

Two Spirit people grow up in everyday families but are somehow different. This experience gives them intimate knowledge of women's and men's ways, yet also of standing apart and being something that includes yet is also beyond both. In western spaces gay and lesbian is often considered just different. The labels separate people. In native cultures we draw people together. We find our common pathways. We are after all a family, a people.

Therefore, over the years it seems that Mi'kmaq Two Spirit ways suggest a pathway forward in living and manifesting the core ethical values of native spiritual ways. This is a powerful realisation and gives some purpose to Two Spirit youth today who are seeking answers as to why they are who they are. This gives youth who are questioning their gender and sexuality a way to explore deeper meanings than are currently available. For those who are struggling with being different and who maybe have lost hope and are even contemplating self-harm or suicide, the teachings in this book are not easy to follow but they actually give hope. There is a way forward. You are made good. You have a place, a purpose, and even a destiny. My mother had a way of telling me this all of my growing years and into adulthood. You have a purpose. You will do something great one day. You will find your path. She said these things so many times, and I often wondered why. Perhaps I will never know why. But her way taught me that youth need to hear this message again and again.

Youth today need a positive and deeply spiritual purpose. So here it is. Males have a purpose and a destiny. You just need to step onto this path and start learning. Women have a profound medicine and power. You only need to awaken to this truth now and start living within your inner voice, your inner power.

The Mi'kmaq Two Spirit path is spiritually available to everyone. No wonder. We Two Spirits are called to integrate men's and women's medicine plus to walk this new way of being. The path is about learning and growing and then sharing your teachings with others. Not on a soap box or from a branch of a tree. Teaching is about living in loving committed friendships and in family. We admire this pathway in the family of Kluskap, who is the first student of the Mi'kmaq Two Spirit Nation. Every youth is Kluskap learning to relate to body, self, others, and creation. As you accept you are Two Spirit in nature, you step on the path. The rest will follow. Stay calm. Breathe deeply. Dance like there is no tomorrow.

Walking the spiritual Red Road to personal power and freedom takes guts and commitment. All you need to do is say 'yes.' Let life do the rest for you. There are lessons to learn and many challenges ahead. There is reward. We have a purpose in life. We have roles and purpose in our culture. In the wider society we can take on many leadership roles we never thought possible.

Many Two Spirit youth awaken through similar pathways. Growing up alone, feeling isolated or different, can lead to deeper suffering. Perhaps also acting out in ways that can be self-harming or cause others grief. This is why having knowledge about the Two Spirit nature provides good teachings and options to help everyone understand human growth and cultural ways. Spiritual emergence can cause crisis. For example, dreams can be very confronting and open new awareness we are not ready for yet. Dreams can come to teach a Two Spirit youth about other people and their sorrows. A wide range of strange experiences can lead a person who is new to this path to feel even more alone and confused.

Confusion may lead you to search far and wide for answers or to shut down and become cynical. Hopefully you choose to stay open and learning. As you begin to accept yourself just a little bit more, the experiences may fascinate you and lead to learning, observing, and seeing what new mystery is around the corner. New pathways open up for people when we listen and learn.

Eventually this capacity of a man to love men becomes a great gift to be cherished. The gift of a woman to love other women is something beautiful. From childhood or young adult sadness a most profound joy comes into the heart when you allow love to be possible. But this needed to be learned again and again. Your depth of pain is directly part of your capacity to love. You have loved so very deeply. Your love is deep and abiding. Two Spirit capacity and abilities are highly prized by many people. It is a wonder how gifts and talents can be celebrated when you least expect.

Depression - This Too Will Pass

One of the most important things to realize when we are young, frustrated and impatient is that everything we feel will not last forever. No feeling lasts for long. Even a deep depression has its shades of grey and blue and different tints of black. Even in the deepest depressions of youth a spiritual awareness can keep you going. I share this here because the dangers of suicide dramatically increase for Aboriginal youth, then increase again for gay, lesbian and Two Spirit youth. My heart goes out to youth in all cultures and especially in native communities where suicide is an on-going problem. If you are thinking even remotely in those ways let me say that there are pathways into the future that you have no idea exist right now. There are ways forward that you can't feel when you are in a dark mood. It may not feel like it, but every mood change and every darkness is cast out by the light of the sun.

The lessons learned along the way help us to become stronger and then to help other people. Here is a great secret. Depression is a gift and opens new insight into people's hearts. This knowledge helps us later on in life when we became a friend, partner, parent, teacher, healer, counsellor, and Medicine Two Spirit. We need to learn how to dance with the shadows. We can learn to face the darkness and demons for the sake of people who will come to us for help. Two Spirit people know this very well. They are realistic, very real. No bullshit.

Indeed, the darkness of depression is very much like the World Beneath the Earth taught about in the traditional spiritual teachings of the Mi'kmaq people. As a therapist I learned to teach people how to enter into a depression and then how to walk out of depression, so that when they found themselves there they would also know how to learn whatever they needed and then to move on.

Kluskap did not know why he was in the Mi'kmaw world. In fact, each person he asked how did they come to be in that world? He was curious. He was wanting and needing to hear their stories. He also wanted to know why was he in this world, what was his purpose? These needs within us today are not new. And we have a very rich tradition from which to learn how to live in the Earth World in a good way.

Youth need to understand that all states of being and awareness shift and change over time, and that we are more than what we feel. Youth need to understand that we can become masters of our inner worlds and we can deal with any challenges that come our way. Older spiritual initiation rites provide many of these insights and life-skills. Today we are learning these ways again and with fresh eyes.

Like Kluskap we can stand and face the Rising Sun. We can give thanks for the East, South, West and North. We can look up to the World of the Sky and give thanks for Creator giving us life. We can look downward to the Earth Mother and offer gratitude for our bodies given to us from the Sacred Red Sands of the Mi'kmaq Nation. Then finally we can look inward. Here is an amazing learning and awakening. Youth find this absolutely fascinating. We have to discover it ourselves through personal experience.

We look inward, and we become aware of our soul and spirit. Just like Kluskap did. This is our inner being. Our phenomenal energy of being alive. Our soul is the feeling within our hearts, our connections and relationships and all of our thoughts and ideas. Our soul is our relational body. And lives in our solar plexus, which itself is very symbolic because this part of our body which rests just below our stomach is the place of Fire and Light and the Energy of the Sun.

Then Kluskap became aware of his spirit. How profound is that. He connected with his spiritual energy upon awakening from the stone and sands of Mi'kma'ki. Our spirits are the primal life force that we receive from Creator. A part of our essence that can never be destroyed. Our spirit is centred in the tips of our minds inside and above our heads and resides within and around our whole bodies as an orb of Light and Truth. We are beings of Light living for a short time in this skin. The essential energy of our Spirit gives life to our bodies. The truth of this is found when we breathe. Once we stop breathing our Spirit leaves the body and returns to the Spirit World. Kluskap was a very powerful Spirit Being who was given human form from the dirt and sands of the world. We too are given form and our bodies will return to the dirt and sands from which we came. We call this star dust. Because we are the Stars who Sing.

True Nature, True Identity

From these teachings we know that our spiritual being is primary. Our body and gender are important and valued. Our native identity is even more. As we get older our identity changes. This is true for Two Spirit ways just as much as for men and women.

During a time of life, Two Spirit identity may give insights about being both female and male in one body. At times or later in life, identity becomes more kin with totemic powers like Kitpu and Paq'tism, Eagle and Wolf. Two Spirits of Power and others come to influence our life in many ways. We cannot begin to say. Their wisdom and insight guide work in this Earth World.

For a Two Spirit there can be days when you may no longer feel two legged. You may feel more like a wolf. Or more like an Eagle. Your spirit sometimes leaves body and goes off with your kinfolk. Body is left behind like an empty shell. Sometimes we wonder if a passage to the next world might not be death, but something quite strange like transforming into an Eagle and flying freely.

Youth need to know that the Two Spirit path is something that can be respected, admired and is way cool. The Two Spirit path is also like its own pathway of mastery and skill. To take this path seriously can lead a person toward the heights and depths of human spiritual and cultural wisdom. Funny how today we are all so busy we do not take time to learn these ways. But life has its own nature. What goes around comes around. Our

Ancestors did not sacrifice their blood and tears for nothing. Their power and wisdom come down to us whether we listen or not. Often times this power seems to cause sickness and illness, upset and mental issues.

Addiction is a powerful twisting of sacred medicines of mind and heart. Addiction is a powerful misuse of sacred medicines of mother earth, like Tobacco and even like the sacred fire water of the Celtic people. Mead was a substance used in sacred ceremony among the Druids. Even today wise elders and a hermit we once sat with know this history and the harm caused by misuse of sacred natural substances that our Ancestors understood were to be used and protected, respected and kept sacred.

There is a good reason why alcohol is called a spirit. Every spirit that gives a gift asks for something in return of equal or greater value. The spirit of alcohol asks a great price, especially for its repeated use, and then its continual use over time. Understanding this is incredibly important. Using alcohol includes the spiritual energy of this exchange. This is often an unspoken agreement or contract. People caught in this shadow covenant or promise first needs to become conscious and aware of the nature of the agreement they entered. But the costs of the exchange often dull our minds to such a degree that once you try to figure things out, the process is triple difficult and the further you go down that road it becomes often near impossible.

We find that for Aboriginal people the teachings on sacred Medicines including with Tobacco, and with the Fire Water of Celtic and European tribes, must be conveyed at times in blunt and direct ways. Otherwise people don't get it. They can waste another ten or thirty years on confusion and painful mistakes for self and family. Creator set things up in a way to give us health and to walk this way of beauty takes guts, determination, and clear thinking. If the nature of substance abuse is spiritual and cultural, then the resolution of addiction is also likely cultural and spiritual in nature. This is partly why many detox programs fail. The underlying spiritual wounds are not healed and resolved. Greater skill is needed by Aboriginal therapists and healers to address these deep and often hidden needs.

Kisiku Sa'qawei Paq'tism takes out sacred Sage and Juniper, places them on the dark coals to smoke and burn and says, M'sit No'kama, M'sit No'kama. Ta'ho.

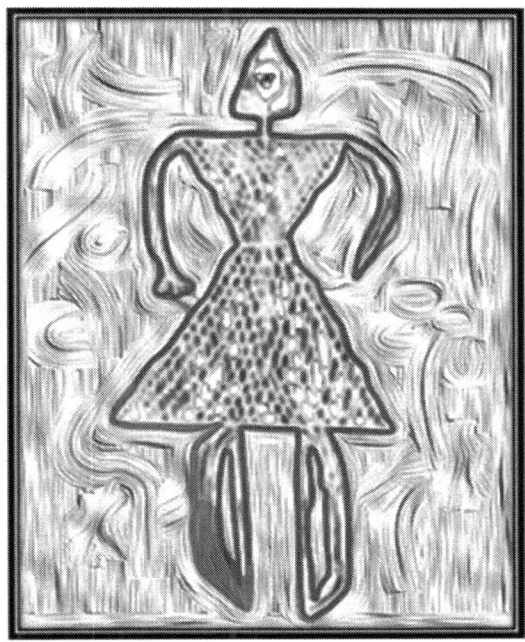

'Some of us are given to the most profound purpose of all. We are called and propelled by our genes, our inner nature. Our hearts were given to us by Creator before we were born. We are impelled into the Sacred Flames of Life to give everything we are to others in loving kindness.'

Two Spirit Oral Tradition

Pjila'si, welcome, come in, sit down. Welcome again. We are L'nu and our nation is strong. This is our sacred fire. This is the Wigwam of Medicine Keepers. Come closer to the sacred fire, be warm and content. Listen now, we have a story to share with you…

Initially and mostly for the sake of Two Spirit people reading this information, as well as for Mi'kmaq people, and for those who wish to support them, including our Metis kin and more distant European cousins, we note that the oral tradition is taken into serious account by ethnographers and historians alike. For scholars examining these issues in future, and for academics, teachers, researchers, health and counselling practitioners, forming reasonable frameworks for practice also ought to allow for the place of oral tradition as a primary source within the construction of knowledge.

We remind readers that within mainstream European and western theory social constructionism holds a great deal of relevance, not simply as a theory but more as a means to explain how knowledge is created and passed on in generational patterns. When backing away from ideology and looking at theory as pragmatic models that help explain phenomena, we come more closely to what I have often documented as principles of Indigenous science. For instance, my work in past has extended the examination of Mi'kmaw ceremonial theory and practice, looking in fair detail at the Medicine Circle and its various layers, components, and means toward healing in emotional and social health and wellness. There is little doubt that native cosmology holds enormous value and teachings for advancing Indigenous and the global human ecological sciences.

To appreciate this cosmology and to understand the primary nature of oral tradition in the creation and passage of knowledge systems, we admit to a model of variance. This model comprises not simply the cognitive ideas spoken in place and time, passed on from elder to elder-in-formation, but also the oral tradition itself supports the variances of and observations to creativity, insight, intuition, vision, and receiving information and wisdom as if from mysterious layers of existence.

These domains or origin-points of knowledge and teachings can be studied and attained in various degrees. The ceremonial path is central to this practice that over time becomes a daily and nightly part of one's life. This forms the ways we look at the world around us, and the means by which we move forward through practice of an Indigenous science of observation, testing ideas or theory, continued observation, analysis and discussion, listening and learning, and over time coming to terms with nature, skill, and agency. Action emerges from an 'elder-based method' of listening with respect common to all ages across the two-legged lifespan.

The Wigwam of Family

The Australian Waradjuri Nation calls this Yindyamarra. The word means to Take it Slow, Listen with Respect, Show Caring in Action. We were honoured to develop a creative art learning and music program for primary school around this Aboriginal teaching.

The action of Yindyamarra is to slow the self-down enough to listen carefully, observe carefully, and proceed with caution in concern for other beings. These principles are kin with Mi'kmaw teachings of the nature of ceremony as life, and life as ceremony.

The Elder gkisedtanamoogk (1993) shares this method of Indigenous learning and seeing through the Wabanaki word Anoqcou. Anoqcou may be translated as 'walking with the star and flower,' as well as sky and earth, cosmos and being, far and near, vision and reflection, knowledge and wisdom. These two poles of the wigwam are joined at the top and extend outward to hold the structure of being, relation, family, tribe, nation. We cannot have one without the other, although we can easily become imbalanced. Around and with these two poles are bound a total of 13 poles that form the wigwam of the family. This sacred circle holds the winter and hearth fire that burns at the centre, in the bones and flesh of Mother Earth.

In fact, the wigwam of family is integral to Mother Earth, not a separate sphere as happens in later colonial western mysticism and Christian cosmology. Fascinating to the study of history is the fact that Indigenous cosmologies tend toward integral methods, and a deep-ecological wisdom. This is also true of the root cultures from which Christianity springs, as well as for the European cosmologies from the Celtic, Druidic, and Goddess paths in those very countries where Christianity came to dominate and replace sacred sites to the Earth Goddess with cathedrals to the demoted Mary of Nazareth.

When you consider the social, emotional, and psychological layers of these teachings you begin to realise the importance of balance, learning, and listening. The point is that 'ceremony as life' as taught by our brother gkisedtanamoogk encourages deeper qualities of being and action that allow people to stay on their path in life, to grow as integral persons.

The diversity and harmony of the wigwam extends to personal awareness in how our many parts come together around the heart fire of gentle strength and growth as a spirit having a human experience. We can see how the depth of these teachings are kin with Two Spirit Medicine teachings. In some respects, the Two Spirit Medicine person often carries solitary practice over very many years, and so advances in degrees within the medicine practice. Again, solitary in the native sense is deeply interwoven, just as the structure of the wigwam's bones and hearth fire are integral to the body of Mother Earth. When we are on our path, we are connected. When we walk with solid ethics, grounded in our loving service, and even when we are not consciously aware, our bodies are part and parcel of the fabric of life, culture, and family – integral to the ecology of all life.

Communication of oral teachings like these arise particularly in regard to contemporary Indigenous research and especially within fields where colonial relations continue to be part of the picture. Professor Marie Battiste made great strides globally and is highly respected in Australia for her efforts in post-colonial research methods and practices in education. Her work inspired me to no end and gave me a clear sense of purpose in both analysis of western mainstream weaknesses and in formulating Indigenous science and practice. On one hand our generations need to examine and deconstruct western theory and practice. This is extremely useful for our purposes. But is also critically important for global and ecological survival of our species on planet earth.

On the other hand, we need to articulate and co-create methods of Indigenous ceremony as research, ceremony as learning, ceremony as teaching, ceremony as therapy, and the exploration of these dynamics, and their circular and spiral logic comprises the curriculum for family life and community education in the coming generations. By basing these models in our cultural traditions, we move forward in post-colonial methods and eventually can drop the notion of colonialism all together and become generative Indigenous sciences and professions in their own right. Even though history suggests the post-colonial framework is essential, because the temptation to disconnect and sever the relations of respect within natural ecology is ever present, and always a danger that needs to be guarded.

The Sacred Pipe of Family

We ought to remember here that in fact the Sacred Pipe Traditions of our people, and the people of Turtle Island and other parts of Mother Earth, has arisen within our ecology for this very purpose – to guard and inspire and instruct. Native teachings, at their core, are entirely ethical and pragmatic. Unlike other ideologies, Native teachings are based in natural science and observation of the interrelations of nature and all life. Truly a science of cosmology, the metaphors and teachings of Native cultural spirituality are not a religion, in the sense of a detached body of philosophy. Once the Native teachings are severed from nature, they no longer exist and become false.

The illogical nature of many colonial beliefs, values, and methods arise precisely because of this mismatch. When the Christian culture ceases to embrace nature, they make grave mistakes that lead to persecution of science, knowledge, and basic human rights and freedoms. The separation from truth is about a severing of natural laws and a rather basic scientific method of observation, listening, humility, and respect that the nature of cosmology is more integral than we can imagine in our limitations today.

Yet the core cosmological feeling or sensation is that wisdom is inherent in the system. This is where we get the lovely metaphor of 'Mother Earth.' There is a sense that life itself has its own wisdom apart from our small ego-view, and when we tap into this larger picture we may not see the forest from the trees. But we can appreciate how the fabric of nature appears to work when we hold respect as primary. The Sacred Pipe Tradition arises from this place.

The Pipe Tradition comes from the sorry business of native familial and community break down. From the severing of relations of respect. The Pipe Tradition arises in the context of ended negotiations, failed treaties, conflict, and war. All of the stories of the origin of this tradition point to the emergence of the feminine White Buffalo Calf Woman or her equivalent. Again, the feminine arises in the two-legged species to voice interwoven connection, the need for really pressing that humility is essential even when we are upset and angry, and that we must somehow pull ourselves back into a mind of connection. The Pipe as a ceremony, as a place and space for changing our minds, is essentially a therapeutic process. The therapy or change needed is changing our minds to a place of listening, being open minded, and willing to place our egos aside to see a bigger picture.

Important to know that the Pipe is the balance of nature. The bowl of the pipe is feminine. The stem of the Pipe is masculine. The combination of stone and wood are deeply symbolic. The stone female bowl is primary, ancient, formed from the first stones of the planet. The wood is temporary, will fade away, be destroyed by fire, and be spent up in smoke as carbon is always recycled in nature. This gives all of us the ethical framework for humility, as the feminine and masculine energies are within all of nature as well. Nurturing and action, carrying and being carried, movement and direction, are integral parts of the spiral of life and they are feminine and masculine in nature.

Our brief discussion about the Sacred Pipe shows how the oral tradition is central and primary to respect of native ways, histories, and teachings. From this you can grasp the importance of this discussion on oral tradition and its right of place in the construction of knowledge. The empowering truth of this remains that we are part of this emerging knowledge field and wisdom practice – right now.

For so long since my youth there was this inner call to solitary life but also to give something essential to others. This quest became clearer when the 7th generation teachings came to our awareness. Then we realised that the spirit within was awakening from ages past. An ancient song was being beaten on the skin of this drum. Solitary life in nature became part of a teaching and learning practice that led to over 200 publications, many books, years of teaching at universities, and years of service as a therapist, founding research journals and professional bodies, and extended retreats in places that allowed medicine practice and freedom to explore life.

But this lifetime started in the very humble places of Nova Scotia and remains humble across many projects and honours. Sitting here writing this now with blankets around this body and the sense of tiredness and cold contrasting the warmth of heart, felt in sharing teachings with you, heart to heart, nothing can be more humbling and levelling. We are all growing older and we will pass away into the spirit world again. What you have now in your hands is your own pathwork. Listen well and carefully, and take it slow with respect. The rest will come to you when your wisdom-time opens space, and options will cross your path you never dreamed possible.

The Meaning of Traditional

We are Two Spirit Mi'kmaq. What else needs to be said? From this place so much learning will be co-created, and so much fun and happiness arise. We can celebrate our lives after eons of shame and fear are gone, but we will always remember.

Two Spirit means a way of loving and caring for each other within community. We are deeply interconnected. We are members of families, tribes and collectives. While discussion of Two Spirit rarely if ever happens publicly, at least during the past, when the issues are discussed people are relatively quick to evaluate personal ethics, boundaries and intentions.

Because of the associations with colonial histories that have distorted culture to such a degree, Two Spirit can often be associated with sex and much like 'gay' in past has been associated with shame and homophobia, similar dynamics can happen with Two Spirit. This is partly why there has been so little mention of Two Spirit in everyday culture, and why the issues are only surfacing in social media and internet sources over the past decade at best.

This is a very recent discussion at this level. Prior to this time, the issues are either largely hidden and silent or discussed among people 'in the know' so to speak. And the deeper knowledge around these issues has not really surfaced and is yet to be revealed in the published literature. In many respects mainstream cultures have not been ready to receive this deeply connected and ecological wisdom. Whenever this wisdom is presented in past, the reasons are distain, disrespect, and outright violence. This is witnessed by history in the simple fact of how the Peace Pipe has been misunderstood and disrespected, and how treaties are overlooked continually and how indigenous knowledge is used and abused by the western academe, science, and political systems.

At the same time, western and colonial cultures are growing and changing, giving rise to greater exchange of knowledge and we hope, awakenings in public opinion that move away from truncated religious biases towards greater open-minded and values based in ecology and spirituality. These changes over the centuries suggest a greater wave of healing and growth among the children of European heritage. For this reason, to a limited degree at least, there is a time of disclosure of certain sacred truths that is coming forward. The Two Spirit Medicine Path is one such body of wisdom that has come of age.

There is no doubt that extended histories of colonial and religions bias play a huge role in these discussions among the Australian, Canadian, New Zealand, and other children of European and Commonwealth families. Among the Commonwealth we share a unique history, and our better-informed USA cousins understand this fairly well even though they chose a different path towards a republic. The European and colonial heritage includes histories of dissociation from sexuality and gender to such an extent because of widespread histories of family violence, sexual abuse, and violations of trust. Religious values in this history have for the most part polarised these beliefs and attitudes, leading to widespread persecution and fear-based policies and practices. Medicine inherited these beliefs and attitudes, and since the 18th century has transplanted bias and prejudice into mental health and illness models that further incarcerated sexual and gender difference.

We should also respect the historical evidence that Mi'kmaq exposure to these cultural assumptions and biases parallels the history of western medicine and science. Our colonial exchange in the main began during the 17th century with French immigration. Therefore, the discussion ought to respect that things take time, and that issues can often be sensitive even today. Talking openly about Two Spirit in today's context is still fairly new and tends to be done only in respected spaces among trusted allies.

At another level there are other issues of trust that arise for young Two Spirit people, and that may include communities and families dealing with former family members struggling with substance abuse and sexual abuse. Where trusting relations are created are compromised and need time for members of families to heal and trust again. It takes patience and honesty. Things will eventually improve particularly because Mi'kmaw culture tends to celebrate healthy human sexuality.

We are seeing across Indian country that Two Spirit cultures can emerge. Projects can be shared. Song Lines and ceremonial patterns can be explored and developed. Internally people are people. Internally Two Spirits on the medicine trail can generate enormous energy for healing, learning, and transformation. These patterns are seen at critical turns of social developments. They give rise to 7th generation prayers and gifts that make a real difference across time and space. And Two Spirit is not about roles and expectations as much as sharing joy and laughter, friendship and companionship, tears of sorrow and deep abiding joy.

Likewise, non-Two Spirit people are quite open to discuss the topic and its issues. Once the ground is cleared of issues of potential selfishness, harm, and abuse by people who might wish to use the Two Spirit platform as a way to manipulate others and possibly the youth of the community, there is great potential for development of Two Spirit teachings. It is important to not allow violations to dominate and prevent advances for youth who really need clear spaces of safety and support.

A strong oral tradition exists today regarding the Two Spirit among the Mi'kmaq. Whether this tradition goes back into history and 'pre-history' before contact with Europeans is of less concern to me than many of my contemporaries.

Many today want to base their approach on the authority of ancient traditions. My approach is to encourage healthy respect for our Elders and Ancestors, but there is no need to be dogmatic. We can leave this attitude to the colonial mind.

Easy enough to be tempted by this shiny notion of appealing to tradition. But we do not need to make tradition into a religion. There are already enough religions in the world. For the sake of learning and listening, allow me to clarify what the word traditional means.

'Traditional' does not mean what existed in the past. In fact, who acts on traditional values but people who are alive and kicking today. Traditional is what people feel now, what they believe and wish to convey. They wish their approach, beliefs, behaviour or ethics to come from a traditional form of native living. But do you see them living in a Birch bark wigwam all year? Not likely. Do they live in wooden and metal houses? Probably. So, this word traditional needs flexibility. The word traditional does not mean ancient, historical, or of the past. A traditional lifestyle could well be forward thinking, sustainable, ecological, and futuristic. In many respects when you consider Indigenous science and ecology this is truer than not.

Really important point. So many people, especially native people, discount anything that smacks as traditional. They are busy working to create a new world based in non-traditional lifestyles that are more in sync with the rest of techno global society. Others have said to me, 'I don't have anything to do with traditional ways. I don't believe in ceremony or traditional medicine. It never helped me.' We say fair enough, peace on your path in life. What would you like to share now?

Different strokes, right. There are many reasons why someone decides their approach to things. Not the least of which is that once culture was fractured into conflicting values because of colonial impacts, and once knowledge systems were challenged by contrary teachings from other cultures and religions, Mi'kmaw traditional and ceremonial practices no longer had as much sway in everyday life. It takes time to bring them back in realistic and meaningful ways. A life experience of living in solitary places while engaging in medicine practice in the old ways might be a bit rare and outside the norm for most of our nation, if anyone did a survey as such... But then again, intuition and elder's suggestions tell us that medicine keepers of high regard tend to be rare and far between during any era.

The point is that traditional more than likely means to take a student's learning and listening method all along the journey, because the more you know, the more you awaken to the fact that you know far less than what the ego wants to believe. There is so much more to learn. Our knowledge and experience are always inadequate to the challenges of life each day. Part of the practice is then to let go of anxiety, to find peace. Smudging and smoking ceremony are helpful for this. Making a cup of calming tea is also soulful. A best day for many is making bread, 'Luski' as we say, 'Damper' in Australia. It is pretty much the same, funny enough, a throwback to colonial flour. Yet highly valued.

Oral traditions are in keeping. Native readers will smile and know this is true. But here again, technology and advances in science and culture actually draw people back into ecology and traditional relations of respect.

My teaching and research career took on the responsibility of pointing out the ways that native knowledge systems are corrective of mainstream and European-based systems that have caused the planet great harm. This is the balance that keeps our survival on this planet. The wisdom comes from our traditions, not from mechanistic or economic reductions. The wholistic nature of native culture and spirituality is ripe with wisdom for futuristic lifestyles.

There is much confusion about what these words actually mean. In many respects Indigenous tradition is actually kin with scientific method when grounded in an ethics of ecology and care for creation. There is even more conundrum about ways forward that can actually embody the best of the traditional values of our People. Likewise, looking through the looking glass in reverse, science as a model for traditional methods can be quite practical and helpful to sort through some of the colonial and historical issues facing our people.

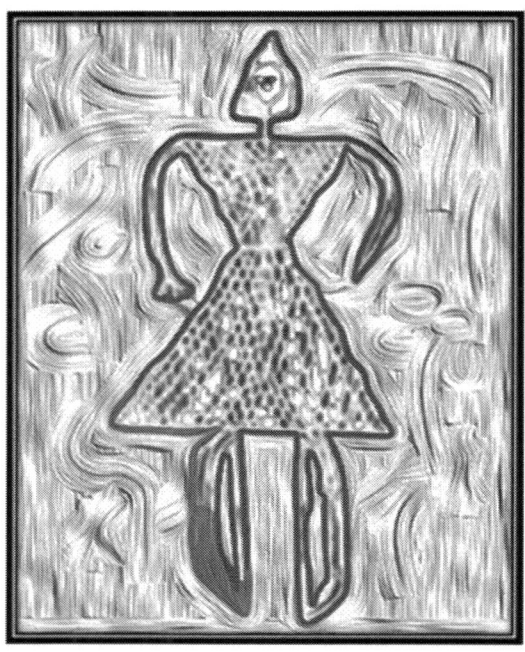

'If we listen long enough and can endure the pain of each other's trauma stories, something beautiful happens. This happened powerfully when we begin to listen to the trauma stories of our Aboriginal friends and family.'

Ambassadors of Memory

Pjila'si, welcome, come in, sit down. Welcome again to our sacred fire. Come closer, stay warm. We can feel the heart opening up, and flowers are blooming everywhere... How rare it is that a child of light awakens. Do not be side tracked by the mind of this age, for in ages past mind was the servant of heart. And the heart was and remains primary. After all, heart holds wisdom and power. Mind is best to follow these ways.

Elders tell me that the Two Spirit, because of their Medicine and Power, were our ambassadors. We have never seen or read this in any accounts. You will very likely never find this written anywhere in the historical record. This is a 'memory' that comes from oral tradition and that several Elders shared. Other Elders confirmed this teaching during our visits to Mi'kma'ki between 2005 to 2010. It is interesting for a number of reasons, because in part we are not aware of direct commentary on an ambassador role generally within the colonial record. The absence of this, and how it was constructed by the colonisers is likely based in presumption and prejudice. That the Mi'kmaq in some way hold the value of national representation even in general terms dating back to first contact and beyond is actually not at all surprising. That this fact remains overlooked in discourse and international political relations between Canada and Mi'kma'ki to this day is incredibly disturbing. But we need to remember that the Mi'kmaq Nation was engaged in international trade, political agreements, confederacies, and strategic alliances long before European contact.

Elders from across Mi'kma'ki from Eskasoni south to Wildcat and Bear River further discussed with me that they feel the Two Spirit were likely among the first people elected to greet the flouting islands and to welcome the first white man who stepped upon the shores of Mi'kma'ki and thus Turtle Island (North America). They recall providing food and especially sacred herbs to the men sick with scurvy, an act of kindness that allowed the first visitors to survive that first winter, was attributed in this way to the Two Spirit who carried the sacred Medicine of herbal knowledge.

Initially and at face value, without any historical evidence per se there is simply no way to confirm or deny these accounts. However, from a cultural view there are several layers of native ways of knowing within the ecology of our understanding that need to be acknowledged. This story of first contact from a Mi'kmaw perspective is astounding if taken literally. And yet the story is plausible if understood in a balanced perspective and taken within the overall oral tradition.

Initially, we must say that there have rarely if ever been comprehensive written accounts from a Mi'kmaw study of the history before Elder Dr Daniel Paul's historical research during our generation. Consider for a moment the implications of this statement. This bears considerable reflection on the entrenched socio-political climate as well as the challenges for a minority culture to address the intractable nature of colonization.

At the same time, we agree that from a purely factual historical perspective to attribute Two Spirit roles, involvement, and official status within Mi'kmaw history may be viewed by some as plausible or felt by others as entirely fabrication. We recall Elder Dr Paul's comments that the field of historiography suggests that all history is an exercise in fabrication, in as much as to create a fabric requires reconstructing existing elements to make something new. That new product is our historical perspective, which historiography suggests is changed in various ways in every generation. That every generation more or less socially constructs history is commonly understood in scholarship and social commentary, even while upholding the value of staying clear on what constitute the facts of history. But even this is hotly contested. As they say, history is written by the victor. Though today, this field is being rewritten by a range of voices.

Looking Back, Looking Forward

However, this is not to say that anyone including the Elders sharing this story can simply accept without question this very interesting comment on Mi'kmaq-European first contact. It could go without saying that there appears to be a sense in which stories carry symbolic power and open up new possibilities in perspective. This instructive and inspiring layer is central to native story telling. Facts and truth per se are not the primary objective, not at least in how the cognitive mind wants to limit both to a concrete reduction. Concrete reduction was not part of traditional native experience in this sense. And is not part of the ways that many native people think and feel about the worlds.

For a number of reasons, the plausibility of an ambassadorial role that was entirely overlooked and/or suppressed in the historical record is worth considering. Certainly, within the historical mention of native representation, even during treaty negotiations, it is equally plausible that the distain felt by European commentators, governors, priests, bishops, military leaders, would be guided by underlying biased and preconceived values. That any given community would send representatives to meet newcomers is also completely understandable. That any given Chief or a chosen representative, and one of the community's Medicine Keepers might be among them is also plausible.

To suggest that any of these characters involved in ambassadorial roles may have been Two Spirit may also be plausible when we consider the logic of this idea from a native perspective. It is not farfetched to think that the community may have intuitively and naturally chosen a person of high degree who may have been of Two Spirit nature to play a role of meeting strangers from another nation. This seems more plausible when there was the need for medical diagnosis and treatment of the sickness of the European men carried during that first winter. That certain Elders may align herbal and medical practice with Two Spirit roles is also plausible, given that these gifts of capacity seem to be part of the Puoinaq role. As hard as this claim of Two Spirit involvement in first contact may be to accept from within current dominant social values, the story may be plausible though can never be proven one way or other.

Let's take this idea at face value. The next question is let's assume for a moment that two foreign cultural differences where meeting for the first time. Imperial European hypermasculinity meets what they view as Mi'kmaq savagery in part due to their perceptions of an absence of Eurocentric gendered norms among the natives. First impressions may have been confirmed by the British view of family structure, family values, and in the treatment of women, children, and elderly.

Had Two Spirit warriors been among the ranks of the Mi'kmaq the best guess today is that they would not have stood out very much. For one, the lack of polarised gendered norms among the Mi'kmaq made the playing field fairly equilateral such that any given person drawn to one or the other feminine or masculine energy would not have had as far to stretch or jump, as it were. As these energies were integral to each other, gender was not constructed per se, but was part of the natural order within a creative focus on personal and social agency. This reading of the history is helpful because the line of reasoning suggests another reason why the Two Spirit phenomenon may not appear in the written records.

It would therefore be quite useful for future generations of Mi'kmaw scholarship to examine the gender relations of our history compared to other native nations where Two Spirit are raised in their historical records. Perhaps for example where in situations where there are accounts written, we suspect that the gender construction of the culture was generally more differentiated and/or polarised than in the Mi'kmaw culture. Perhaps polarisation of gender is a necessary dimension of a culture where Two Spirit roles are tied to more overt expressions of gender, i.e. in dress, conduct and gender-based roles. In other words, the field of discourse may be imposing on Mi'kmaq culture a foreign construct that bears little meaning in traditional pre-contact culture. However, virtually all analysis that exists thus far highlights the negative, and little adequate work has been done to suggest what the Mi'kmaq cultural landscape reveals that is quite independent and distinct from gendered ways of understanding ecology and human life.

It is impossible to believe that this generative work is rendered impossible simply because of the historical contexts of colonization over the past 500+ years. Rather we are convinced that the current reawakening of native culture will indeed nurture the ecology necessary to create future perspectives from within a revived Mi'kmaw cultural practice. This work can then circle back into analysis and reflection on pre-contact cultural ways.

It also stands to reason that the spiritual gifts and capacities of the Puoinaq could have resided in anyone and may not stand out upon first glance. Even when a man was dressed like a woman or woman dressed like a man, if style of dress was all that different to begin with, on initial encounter that person may not have stood out from the crowd. We have discussed style of dress in other places in this book, but we again mention that for a forest dwelling and Canadian winter surviving people, the Mi'kmaq were first and foremost pragmatic. In many ways, dress takes on pragmatic necessities over and above ornamentation. Additionally, and generally, the traditional Mi'kmaq aligned with the birds of the air and other creatures that rendered the male of the species the more colourful. Where European gendered constructions relied on hetero-masculinity as the defining quality, the Mi'kmaq Two Spirit masculine male-skin would not have stood out from the crowd. The Two Spirit feminine male-skin would have been easily overlooked among the women, whose pragmatic dress codes would have been generally understated and quite practical except perhaps during summer gatherings or other special events.

From Plausible to Instructive

How strange those early encounters must have been for our Two Spirited Ancestors. Instead of thinking about the material appearance of those strangers in their European military coats of wool and metal sticks that made huge cracking sounds, our spiritual Two Spirit Ancestors may have looked into these bodies to see their spirits. They would have been dismayed to see that the European was for the most part a mere child.

Respectfully, and from a contemporary psychological analysis, for the majority of men that stepped off the boats the spiritual evolution of the European traveller at the time of first contact was that of a traumatised child, perhaps stubborn and obstinate, and within a polarised personality that fluctuated between externalising authority verses asserting a limited exercise of power within a materialistic worldview. The European that came to Mi'kma'ki and claimed this land for their King never or rarely had the opportunity to grow into their own power, insight, or wisdom. They lived under warlords, and entitled overlords, in a military and monarch state that was dominated by a church-based culture run by clerics and bishops, where women were subservient and owned by men, and where slavery was the norm.

By comparison, the Mi'kmaq had a decentralised culture of leadership based in a highly evolved democratic consensus-based political and social system, governed by consensus-elected chiefs, and served by medicine craft and wood craft among families. Their land sharing was also evolved, and maintained by regional, inter-tribal, and international treaties and advanced confederations. There was no indentured service nor slavery. Women were considered the First Medicine and so held equal status as citizens and exercised leadership positions as well as social and political power among the people.

Respectfully, as many if not most Mi'kmaw families today carry European names and have European ancestors, of our European ancestors their culture had replaced rich Indigenous spiritual traditions with a religious myth based on fear and suppression. They lived within an unbalanced and crude warrior power that was based on abstract dissociated concepts of power, and in a relatively speaking flat-land cosmology that objectified divinity in a monotheistic framework.

In contrast, our families have retained First Nation identity and from this basis our Native cosmology suggests that real power lies within; and is found through self-giving and love. True power is ecological and connective in nature. Only in recent decades is this ecological value system becoming mainstream and global. In part due to Eurocentric values that lead to eco-genocide and environmental crisis.

True of both French and English migrants, the power the men of the flouting islands carried was projected powerlessness, learned helplessness, and submission to external authority. Their learned powerlessness kept them under control and oppression. This is why they never or rarely grew up to be men in the spiritual ways this book conveys. In their conquest they carried guns just as much as they carried the dark medicine of greed, lust, envy, jealousy, and ego-based pride. These values made them appear like lost children to our Ancestors. And where these Ancestors may have been Two Spirit the observation is even more poignant. No wonder those first visitors appeared lost to the first generation of Elders faced with colonial contact.

The spiritually adept of our People, perhaps our Two Spirit Ancestors may have stood on the shores of the great lake, and they may have witnessed a coldness of heart. Perhaps they laughed, maybe they shuddered. This must have influenced the perception that these newcomers were quite harmless. Like children who had never been taught the ways of a civilised society. This perception may have come from how the Two Spirit could have witnessed the newcomer's spiritual immaturity, their lack of practical knowledge for survival, and their frailty and lack of health. But how much more dangerous is an immature people who carry firearms and weapons of ecological destruction that were inconceivable to the first contact Mi'kmaq.

Could it be true that the Two Spirit warrior and Medicine Keeper reached out to the dying men and cured their scurvy with the cleansing drink of our forests? We may never know. But raising the question holds a powerful poetry and irony that only the Mi'kmaq can fully appreciate. We can remember in this sacred way how these Two Spirit Elders sought out the sacred herb, boiling it up, and shared it among the dying men from across the great pond.

It may also have been observed by our Two Spirit Ancestors how the newcomer's tribes generally treated one another with a lack of respect, with fear in their eyes, and with the desire to escape oppression. Over the years some of those men defected and joined our Indian Nation. These men were like the political refugees of today who wish to escape the oppressive culture of their origins.

It was also observed how the European spiritual leaders generally instilled fear and did not inspire love or genuine respect. Perhaps less so among the French, these ways of the newcomer's tribe were well known. The newcomer's military culture did not inspire as much as demand respect, did not instil admiration as much as fear. Even while the resourcefulness of the flouting islands and the implements and technologies of the newcomers were of great interest, they also proved to be destructive. Their usefulness was quickly overshadowed by the greed and selfishness of the invader. Perhaps many of our Elders would not touch these implements because of the negative energy they carried. The crude physical manifestations of technology were of no concern to the spiritual ones among our Ancestors.

After all, what good is a knife or a gun when they are used to kill another man for the sake of a bottle of rum? We learned early on that the white man's technology comes with a cost that is very high. We learned early on that the European people carried an underlying cultural and spiritual void that allowed these behaviours to go unchecked. This may have caused our Two Spirit Ancestor great concern, because they had never encountered friend or enemy who walked with a sleeping spirit like the newcomers. Great technological power in the hands of a child is dangerous. We learned to observe and be cautious. This attitude has continued down through the generations.

In relation to the history about to unfold, these early impressions did not awaken sufficient resistance to the newcomers fast enough. There was a time when the Mi'kmaq population was large and strong. When they had the political strength to expel the newcomers or to at least create greater leverage for later negotiations. Instead the first generations during colonial contact took pity on the newcomers and welcomed them into the Earth World of the Mi'kmaq, much to the eventual demise of the Aboriginal Nations of Turtle Island.

Ancestral Memory and Recovery

Now fourteen generations from our first French Acadian forefather who lived during the mid 17th century, the heart feels the responsibility of this knowledge like a profound weight of sadness and determination. Reflecting on this history, it is not without reason that the invaders among the French and the British may have, for different but similar reasons, sought to first attack the integrity of the spiritual leadership among the people. Naturally we surmise that there may have been Two Spirit among our leaders in herbal lore, medicine practice, ceremony, men's and women's business, and keeping memory of who could marry who to maintain healthy families. These and many varied skills and talents were shared by the people.

It seems plausible that the early priests may have overlooked if not attacked the Medicine Keepers because they represented the spiritual core of the Nation, that which the invader could not understand beyond their conceptions of witchcraft or sorcery. The Puoinaq were very likely looked at in this light from the earliest days of French-Mi'kmaq contact. Under British authority the dynamics shifted away from domestic collegiality into outright conflict and war. Discussing subtle differences was no longer part of the discourse. Extermination was on the table and became the operational motive. As the history shows, we were savages in their eyes.

The fact of history is that human rights were largely unknown by the colonial machine. Christianity was also governed by imperial and corporate Roman values translated into feudal monarchies that remained well into the modern era. The system was based on conquest objectives that sought to control, own, and destroy the forests for their ships; the seas for their fish; and the people for their audacity to stand in the way of progress.

The colonial invasion inside European nations themselves is important to understand. This process was psychological as much as physical for everyone involved in the already centuries old transformation of Indigenous European cultures into colonial powers. The dominant values that came to define colonialism are linked to a philosophy that had become dissociated from natural and human ecology since before the Roman invasion of Britain. People today are dealing with many of the very same underlying value conflicts when addressing the modern political economy, global monetary systems, and issues such as deforestation, extinction of species, degradation of the environment, climate change, and global warming.

Remember our discussion about women being demonised and burned as witches. This was among the traditions of how the newcomers of British influence treated women. Again, the first contact with the Mi'kmaq was mostly with the French who had a slightly more relaxed perspective on women's roles. French views of masculinity were a bit more flexible than the British. This was in part why the French respected or at least feigned respect of the Mi'kmaq Nation.

On the other hand, the colonial British were the skin-heads of the era. The historical record clearly shows the British could be compared to the Nazi who engaged in ethnic cleansing and genocide so that their own race would rise above all the rest. They raped and pillaged without respect. The details of the history of their treatment of the Mi'kmaq are shocking to recall, and this history is well documented in official records that cannot be disputed.

The British of the era were terribly repressed. They treated women, children, and the elderly with coldness. These values were internalised by women in their culture. Children were to be seen, not heard. Women would impart their knowledge in silent ways for fear of men's anger. While realising these values and behaviours, you will also tune into how the Europeans felt about spirituality, family life, raising children, and about issues of social justice.

The fear-based and oppressive materialism of the European psyche of the 17th and 18th century relied on the right of kings to rule by black gun powder. This crude militaristic state governed human relations, and their religious worldviews supported the notion that people must dominate and subjugate creation. The myth that democracy came from Britain is indeed a work of folklore. Likewise, the God of the newcomers was largely a vengeful dictator whose son Se'sus came to liberate the human spirit, but whose priests and ministers largely stood by and condoned human slaughter and untold suffering.

In comparison the Mi'kmaq Nation of the 17th century demonstrated an advanced form of democracy through the governance of local councils, regional councils, and larger inter-tribal confederacies. To be fair tribal life was not devoid of fear or the exercise of power. However, the emphasis in the culture was on time honoured values of respect for each person's innate Creator-given authority.

In this way, children were placed at the heart of the Nation and given great respect and latitude. Because children learn what they live, the youth of the culture knew their traditions well. They respected their Elders because they were also shown deep respect in their childhood. What was given, came around. In many respects these ancient Mi'kmaw teachings on child development and parenting appear today in some of the best models of psychology, social work, and education. Likewise, for the Mi'kmaw women were respected as equals. But even this idea of modern-day 'equality' cannot compare to the rightful place of women in Mi'kmaw society. We must press further to understand the sacred place of women in the Creator's original design.

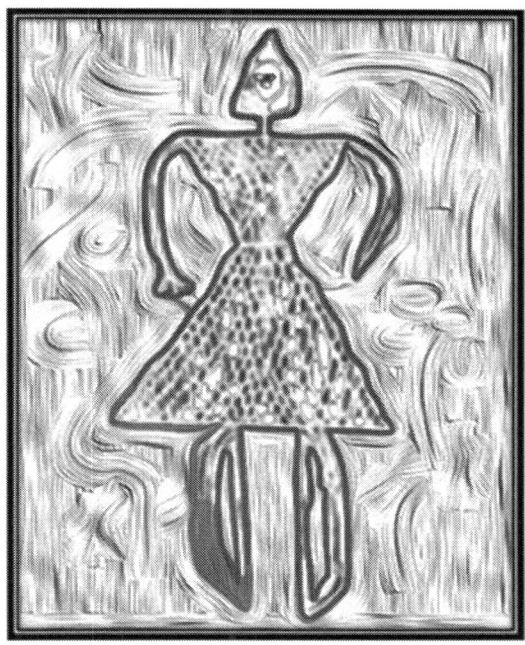

'I can remember… seeing a Great Grandmother in traditional dress, she was weeping and singing out to her grandchildren generations down the line. Then it hit me. She might be singing to us so one day we might wake up and remember who we are… When you realise this, life is changed forever.'

Two Spirit Gender Deconstruction

Pjila'si, welcome, come in, sit down. Welcome again to our sacred fire. Come closer, stay warm. Come in out of the deep cold of winter. There is a fire here that heats the heart and mind with memory, smiles, and laughter.

The Two Spirit way suggests that women, and especially our Grandmothers, are indeed at the heart of the Nation. It was the greatest honour for the Two Spirit male-bodied to serve the Grandmothers, and to assist the younger women on their moon time. The men of the Nation upheld the Two Spirit as great spiritual and practical helpers, extremely valuable to the tribe. This was not because of the skill of the Two Spirit individually. This was based on the respect for Women's Medicine being the First Medicine from which all people come.

Again, these teachings will be disputed and debated, and many will say they have no historical validity whatsoever. In all fairness, to say this may disregard the centrality of oral tradition. The reason why these stories are shared here is not to claim historical 'truth' per se, but to point a way forward in metaphor and narrative with a sense of integrity for the well-being of people today. These are actually stories of our survival and our cultural revival. As such there is a balance of values in a circle of values that places an historical heart-felt respect alongside a self-discerned cultural reflection on our past, present, and future as a people. This is a therapeutic process and ought to be empowering and uplifting.

To uphold women's sacred place among the people is to gain strength and to set a path toward healing, education, and social development. There is an actual therapeutic and social value to many of the claims in this book that are based in ethical and ecological principles. The insights may hold quite old seeds of hope and values that inspire courage, and that need to replant in today's family life. Elders say that our Ancestors are surely living in the next World and will help us understand and appreciate these teachings.

It could be that a male-bodied Two Spirit of high spiritual degrees was taken into women's Medicine, entrusted much like a modern day 'doctor' to care for women during their moon time, or when they were ill, or dealing with physical challenges. In other words, what people do is not who people are. Being male-bodied might be part of who a person is, but from the Native view what the person does cannot be confused with body per se. The two are like comparing the nature of an Ash tree with the fact that many trees have leaves or needles. One suggests an identification of a species of tree, the other is about the nature of many trees and trees in general. Being of a male-body or female-body expresses whole groups of trees but really tells us very little about the nature of the person and their spirit that inhabits the body.

In this sense, gender as we see things in the modern world is obtuse, crude, and reductive. Modern gender theory cannot adequately hold the rich cultural deposit of Mi'kmaw cosmology. In the older traditional cultural sense, and not unique to the First Nations, identity rests in metaphors of relationships rather than in an objectified definition and so this inner sense of identity actually shifts, changes, grows, and manifests differently - even over one's lifetime. Hence to speak of gender does a disservice in one sense, even while the idea of gender today provides a generic and global-type meaning to the nature of all trees, so to speak.

Likewise, a gifted healer can arise in the community in any form, with any range of (non)gendered or sexual identity characteristics. We cannot easily apply the rather boxed-in labels we use today to describe and understand the past, especially within another culture. We Mi'kmaq can be humble enough to remind ourselves that the past is like a foreign country. We are not such gifted seers to know exactly how people lived and what they believed in a time before our time.

Yet our traditional beliefs are quite dynamic. Experience of life has taught me that the Sacred Medicine and Dreaming are not dead and can be revived by people today. This does not make for a complete cultural reconstruction, because we are not willing to impose experiences and beliefs on the past. We can be quite prepared to take responsibility for our beliefs today as reflecting personal lived experience. We can admit life today may have an arm's length relationship with the historical past, or what little we actually know about that past. This connection of arms-length relation with the past is actually about respect for many Native people. This remains closely connected to our heart.

In our experience of women's Medicine, the First Medicine, Mother Earth Medicine, we acknowledge the ancient and enduring power of the spiritual and temporal laws that govern the universe of the Mi'kmaq – and all people of this planet. This Medicine holds the origins and methods of the sacred elements of earth, wind, fire, and water. But for you to know this, you need to actually practice the Medicine Ceremonies. You need to live in the sacred circle during seasonal times, and during sunrise ceremony. You need to stand by your Elder Grandmother holding her Ancient Sea Turtle Medicine Shell that was handed down from generation to generation in her family line, given when the time was right to the next Grandmother of the line whose task was to carry this Sacred Gift and Responsibility. You cannot judge these teachings until you live them in some way.

These elements or ecologies are Living Beings who influence our lives even today, especially today. We ignore these laws to our own demise. These teachings are not foreign to contemporary ecological sciences, which study the wholistic ways of our culture to gain new insights that move beyond the limited worldviews of the past generations of European traditions.

We ought to acknowledge that the dignity of the Mi'kmaq Two Spirit rests on the inherent dignity of women. This is also true of the woman Two Spirit, whose path may be to embrace male Medicine teachings and practices. Yet also true many of the female-bodied Two Spirit explore another layer of the feminine arts and provide another Gift to the people, both to men and women of the nation.

Now if you place all these ideas together, you will realise exactly why the newcomer on Mi'kmaw soil have taken so long to understand and respect the deeply spiritual ways of our People. The European was threatened by the Mi'kmaq Nation's way of life precisely because of how we respected Women's Medicine, children's rightful place at the centre of culture and life, and the highly important place of Elders among our People.

If you look at these three members of the European family these are the very ones who have gained all the attention in western social movements over the past few centuries and decades. But don't expect mainstream people to give Native people any credit, even though we have often been the lone witnesses to equality and ethics over the past 500 years.

With these insights we have shared it should be no surprise how threatening the Aboriginal culture was to the men who walked off their flouting islands. They saw 'savages' precisely because women, children, and elder Grandmothers were at the heart of the Nation. To their feeble minds this could only mean an inferior people. Because in their cultural way, women, children, and the elderly were expendable commodities. Women were sold on the slave trade, bought through contracts of marriage, and used as pawns of governors, kings, and despots. They could not possibly understand that the complex cultural web of Mi'kmaw society linked the roles of women, children, and elders within a profound law of respect within a wholistic cosmology and spiritual way of life. Most did not look long enough to learn of the written language of the Mi'kmaq, nor did they see the regional and socio-political systems in place for governance and land usage.

Song Lines and Medicine Trails

This leads me to conclude that today's youth and adults are setting a pathway forward with integrity and justice in mind for Two Spirit youth. Because of the contemporary evolution of the Two Spirit movement across the tribes of North America, today there is a growing and vibrant community who identify as Mi'kmaq Two Spirit. This is a new and exciting time for many. We are reviving the tribe and bringing home the Medicines. We are awakening what feels like ancient Song Lines, dances, and teachings that bring forward age-old visions of how we wish to live in peace and harmony.

In the contemporary Two Spirit Mi'kmaw body rests the blood of many nations. These bloodlines sing out for reconciliation. This Song Line is sung with Sacred Medicine Pipe during this 14th generation. This is the White Moose Medicine Path given birth among us during these times.

Like many of our cousins and many our age, this 14th generation carries a deep disquiet. On one hand we are disturbed by the memories of injustice done by the wars of the past that created this fragile country of Canada. It may be that today we seek a new path that honours and respects native rights, regardless of the implications to national systems and corporate interests.

On the other hand, people today are more informed. Information technology assists and social media allows people to share the facts about our history. New forms of social and political governance need to rely on all forms of information, all cultures ought to be part of this dialogue. And clearly Indigenous cultures have the most to offer of all world cultures simply because our connections to the land and sea are entirely oriented toward sustainability.

We all, regardless our origins, have within our bodies a rather strong genetic memory of justice. It is not rocket science to see these past colonial wrong doings that are sustained and repeated by today's Indian Act in Canada, and by corporate decisions and policies, and by the Australian governmental approaches to land rights and employment. Social welfare systems in Australia, Canada, and other commonwealth nations are still governed by anti-Indigenous values. Children are still taken out of Indigenous communities, disconnected from their culture and extended families. How can anyone allow this to continue?

No doubt that we all carry in our body the pain of the past fourteen generations of colonisation. All people must awaken to acknowledge that these patterns relate to our mental health and well-being. We must acknowledge that unless we do something now, our children and grandchildren will continue to carry these injustices in the form of sickness and spiritual crisis.

Now is the time to awaken. We call upon the Four Sacred Directions. In Power we Raise the Sacred Mi'kmaq Nation Pipe and call upon Kitpu L'nuinpisun, Eagle with the Medicine. We send forth the Sacred Smoke to the Eastern Door, before the Rising of Dawn, when all the People still sleep. We pray for Spirits of Light to be Strong. As Mi'kmaq Medicine Keepers we bring the integrity of our Lives Today into the Sacred Circle. As Two Spirit People with Medicine we Walk Home. We stand in Unity with Ancestors whose Spirits are Strong and Sure. We are one People. Regardless our differences. We are Mi'kmaq. L'nuk. The People. Stand with us.

M'sit No'kama - All My Relations

Pjila'si, welcome, come in, sit down. Welcome again to our sacred fire. Come closer, stay warm. Many grow weary in the cold winter, and many come to the fire for warmth. This is a natural part of human life. We need one another to stay healthy. We two-legged need the trees, and wood of the fire, more than any tree needs our help. This teaches respect.

Whitehead's (2002, pp. 148-152) book recounts the medicine tales of Jerry Lonecloud. As just one example of fragments of Two Spirit wisdom that may remain hidden within the ancient stories of our people, this short clip from one of Lonecloud's tales provides a wealth of untapped possibilities. Reading and listening to the stories of our people can reawaken hearts and provide parched minds with nourishment.

Lonecloud says that 'Kluskap was a doctor or a medicine man, and he grew his medicine in his garden. Kluscap was great with all things, but a great medicine man…' We have known a few medicine keepers in our lifetime who have taught us many things about the value of herbal lore. The thirst for experiential knowledge of growing and tending plants has been a great inspiration over the years and led to exploring eastern Canadian and Australian herbal wisdom.

The link between Kluscap as cultural hero, medicine keeper, and herbalist are important when understanding the Puoinaq Two Spirit phenomena. In many ways, these lessons provide the skills necessary for transformative action.

In Lonecloud's words, there were 'five great warriors' who 'went on to see Kluscap.' The number five may seem important as the associations are many, including with the five points of the human body. The men in the tale may represent the complete diversity of humanity.

Also significant, Lonecloud suggests that, 'This is the last time Kluscap was seen by the Mi'kmaq…' This implies the importance of the tale to some degree, if not to also suggest that the age of Kluscap had somehow come to an end. Something we Mi'kmaq people may one day challenge.

As the men spoke their wish, Kluscap imagined ways to accomplish. One man was named Ksu'skw. Lonecloud says that, 'Kluscap took Ksu'skw out of his camp and stood him alongside of Nimoqinuk. Ksu'skw became a hemlock tree' (Whitehead 2002, pp. 148-152).

Quite beside the fact that the male identified in Lonecloud's last tale of Kluscap holds a gender variant name with the suffix 'skw' meaning woman, the more telling layers of the story recall the meanings associated with the Eastern Hemlock tree. Kluscap being identified by Lonecloud as a great herbalist and Medicine Keeper is significant. Clearly there may be important lessons to be learned from study of herbal wisdom. From many other sources including our memory of learning herbal lore over the years, Hemlock holds a particularly powerful place among the trees of Mi'kma'ki or eastern Canada.

Hemlock was commonly used to line beds for sleeping on the bare earth as it provided a great deal of warmth in the wigwam. Hemlock was also used to line the walls of the wigwam. Hemlock bark is named in other Mi'kmaq tales as providing good heat in the fire. These meanings suggest that the full embrace of the Hemlock provided the Mi'kmaq with a great deal of warmth. Hemlock tea is also of common usage, as it provides for high quantities of vitamin C and allows one to overcome the cold. Thus, the herb was used internally as well as externally in a number of ways.

As the story provides only male warriors, one of the hidden meanings might be homosocial. Keeping warm at night may then be associated with Ksu'skw which is a curious if not funny allusion. Likewise, Hemlock is associated with magical properties of transformation. One story from memory is associated with Water Fairies who could change into Weasels and into the brides of Stars.

The Hemlock is mentioned as a kind of World Tree by which Spirits move between the World of the Stars to the Earth World. The Hemlock needle kept in one's personal Medicine Pouch or pocket is considered an important talesman and form of magic power. In certain tales singing to the Hemlock needle provides powers of safety, transformation, and regeneration. Again, stories suggest an internal usage, even in vomit arising from the person, suggesting that what is internal becomes external much like taking tea into the body provides a form of change in energy and power.

Naturally we cannot presume to name or know the meanings of the tale from Lonecloud. Nor can these other tales be directly associated with Two Spirit phenomena. And certainly, funny as it seems, the Hemlock tree cannot be directly made into a Two Spirit symbol nor the beginnings of a queer herbal. Equally strange, in all truth the possibilities of metaphor are endless. And in Mi'kmaq traditional ways and medicine stories there are not a few poignant metaphors that are actually intentionally deployed by storytellers to enable youth and others to awaken to new levels of awareness, diverse associations, and creative outcomes that may never have been considered before.

This very epistemology of discovery and celebration of diversity in creation is central to the Mi'kmaq language, storytelling traditions, and cultural values. It is not that farfetched to discern gender and sexuality variant meanings in ancient tales that have, until this time, remained largely limited by colonial heteronormative cultures.

Likewise, the current generation needs to awaken more so to the fact that the storytelling tradition is not part of the past. Stories must be reawakened, reclaimed, and stories will continue to have a life of their own. Every generation is required to give rise to storytellers who continue this spirituality of culture and ecology of metaphor. It just may be that Kluscap will reappear to the people again. Creation of the worlds is not a finished affair, and the ways that we grow are continual and vital.

Story as Medicine

This chapter introduces another sacred medicine story from the Two Spirit tradition. Like all stories of the People, this one arises from ancient teachings and present-day story telling through culturally infused practices.

As a story keeper we seek to reconnect with the truths and metaphors that speak power over the lives of largely marginalized peoples. We find story-keeping kin with medicine-keeping. Both are part of the sacred business. Both give rise to women's knowing and men's knowing.

There are layers of ceremonial specialisations that sometimes overlap and that seek to draw forward harmony, healing, and strength in people's ways of being. Relationships and families are strengthened by these methods. Story is like the work of fire-keepers, because stories warm our hearts. They give the heart inner light and meaning. They show purpose and ways forward. They are a step away from the sacred dreaming of our Ancestors, so can lead us into states of calm, quiet, rest, and sleep. This is healing.

Stories are one of the central methods of helping Two Spirit youth that also need empowerment, recovery, and reawakening. This is why this particular story is so very powerful. And why the sacred word for power and Two Spirit goes hand in hand. An astute counsellor or teacher or helper will use stories in therapy or education or at just that right moment, to not impose an ideology but rather to convey open-ended and deeper meanings that actually allow the youth or person who is seeking to find their own answers. Stories are our medicine.

As for the potency of stories, it cannot be underestimated as to the power of cultural reawakening. But equally potent are the tides of prejudice, racism, violence, colonial values, and the dark side of the politics of gender and sexuality that in fact constitute central interwoven characteristics within the colonial and western cultures. These frames of mind and heart override many of the sacred traditions, sidestep and render minority other ways of knowing, and systematically if not indirectly oppress and condone oppression. This is the nature of western and imperial constitutions that govern everything from church canon law to corporate and civic law.

Central to these systems is the notion of automatically enrolled and the marked absence of opt out. Enrolment in the system is presumed and ratified by the constitutional nature of things. Opt-out as an option is often not provided by this system. Thus, for many individuals, groups, or whole populations and nations, opting out, by the very nature of the constitutional definitions themselves that disallow freedom and human rights, becomes a political, cultural, social, and economic project and a necessity. This option to opt out can be expressed in a multitude of ways, from subtle to overt, from passive social means to full on conflict and war. Yet in the heart of the matter, from our perspective as therapists and educators working across cultures identity is central to universal human rights that are best upheld and respected.

Stories assist in understanding these dynamics of social and political life. Two Spirit people are among the most misunderstood segment of minority populations, carrying double and triple forms of stigma. As such, there is a great confusion about the nature of Two Spirit identity and purpose. This essay seeks to provide a narrative and culturally based form of teaching while allowing the reader to learn from the deeper meanings hidden within the story itself. This is part of our tradition. This is how we learn. A multi-layered approach given to paradox, profound association, and spiritual teaching.

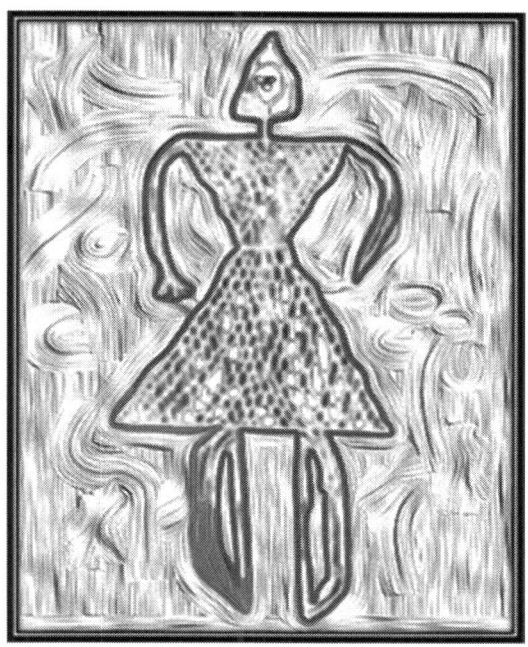

'Human beings naturally move towards healing. We do this because we naturally want to be healthy, well, balanced, and caring spirits. We live in our sacred drums with skin stretched over us… Great Spirit knows who we are and waits for us to awaken… When one human spirit wakes from sleep, every part of creation shivers, sings, and dances.'

A Tale of Two Spirits

Pjila'si, welcome, come in, sit down. Welcome this day to our sacred fire. Come closer, stay warm. Before sharing the story, another tale bears mention. This is again from our dear sister Ruth Holmes Whitehead who we had such a blessing of time and sharing over the years. When we first met her, she was feeling quite sick. But her hospitality was heart-warming, as she spent the afternoon with us well beyond the call of duty.

In one of her accounts that is shared in Stories from the Six Worlds (1988), Ruth transcribes the wisdom of the Horned Serpent being. We feel this story holds particular relevance to the notions of shapeshifting, identity transformation, gender variance, and Two Spirit wisdom. We recommend you get hold of her book, the tales are completely compelling and have become central texts in the Mi'kmaw canon.

She writes, 'There is power in the serpent track, and it begins to change the man. His body thickens and lengthens. He becomes strong and terrible…' The man in the tale had felt for whatever reason to lay down in a strange trench that appeared in the forest. The trench may have been created from an earth quake or other natural phenomena. Perhaps it bore the likeness of a serpent winding through the forest.

Like many Mi'kmaw tales the transformation of a person holds many meanings and happens often. Here the man 'is changing into a jipijka'm himself…' That is, into a Horned Serpent being. He catches the scent of a female serpent being named Jipijka'mi'skw. Horned Serpent Woman. The man 'begins to move in her track, moving in her serpent shape, following her smell down to the water…' Again, movement from earth to water is another form of elemental transformation. Once into the World Beneath the Water, the man seeks out his feminine counterpart.

Meanwhile, back in the land of the two-legged living, Whitehead transcribes that, 'In their camp was a puoin, a shaman, a man whose Power was great…' He was brought into the crisis of identity by the family of the man undergoing such astonishing changes. With effort the shaman determines the outlines of the story and manages an intervention. 'Now the puoin gives medicine to the man taken from the Horned Serpents. It is powerful medicine, and it makes him vomit' (Whitehead, 1988, pp. 44-45). Like in other tales the insides and outsides of a body contain important meanings, connoting changes, transformations, and means to curing or resolving conflicts.

Much like in Jungian psychology, each element of the tale may convey parts of a person, and their interaction relates to aspects of dynamic changes we experience over time. Wisdom teachings are not literal per se. Cultural wisdom describes, or more aptly said, suggests metaphorical associations and multiple meanings within culture. In many respects these meanings can be lost when outside of the mother language of the people. But we have found that even for non-native speakers, the mindset and heartfelt ways of the Mi'kmaq are more important than linguistic dogmatism. Like many elders have suggested, the feeling of the Old Ones of the People is eternal and can be accessed and lived because of its inherent and integral nature.

The tale of the Horned Serpent Male/Female is quite interesting. The horns associated to the female are a masculine image, yet the serpent's winding body ascribed to the male is a feminine connotation. The dangerous changes appear ascribed to a male taken from his female partner, yet he is turned into a feminine dimension who is chasing a female. Then we have a male shaman working with his masculine World Tree or Pole, as often the Medicine Keeper Shaman kept such a large stick outside their Wigwam as an object of power. But the shaman uses feminine aspects to convey an even more feminine soft interior to the male, who vomits up his temporary insides revealing the more stable aspect to his person.

The tale concludes with the warning that had he slept under the blanket of the female serpent or stayed one more night in her Wigwam, he would have been lost among the Horned Serpent nation. One might wonder about the nature of identity changes that require repeated exposure or habits of thought and action.

In some respects where bisexuality is normative within the species, as revealed by modern studies undertaken with the Kinsey Institute since the 1960s, we can easily surmise that the Old Mi'kmaq observed in creation and behaviour how people might shift quickly, and otherwise change over time, towards staying in the camp and wigwams of another family group or gender. Likewise, and as all cultures have tended to conclude throughout history, the capacity of people to 'shapeshift' into new intimate relationships among other types of people is well known. Changes of alliance, sexual affiliations, and identities are clearly part and parcel of the old tales and yet these meanings have not yet been explicitly explored. Naturally the colonial gaze would have prevented this exploration. But future generations of Mi'kmaw youth do have these same constraints. There is more sacred intimate and sexual business ahead for Mi'kmaw youth drawn to understanding the old tales and to uncovering these mysteries.

The section below is an adaptation of a story that was first published under Bowers (2005a). The story was first entitled 'Shieldwolf and the Shadow.' The Shieldwolf was the Scout wolf that went ahead of the pack to look for safe passage and foraging of game. The Shieldwolf doubled back to let the Alpha know what they found, to guide the pack safely. The link also was associated with the author's middle name Randolph, which in Teutonic means Shieldwolf. After many years of having been given by Mi'kmaq Elders the name Paq'tism, these meanings surfaced and provided inspiration for this story. These associations are secondary however. The raw power of the story lies in this current context. We are relieved that the Paq'tism story can be reclaimed from colonial discourse and can finally be set to rest within its natural home within this book. Now onto our Two Spirit story at hand...

Ta'pu Miijaqamijjk Puoinaq Paq'tism

An Elder once said, there was at one time, in the old, old days, a young man who suffered greatly with anger. He felt inside of himself the pull between anger and love. Violence and kindness. The war was so strong this young man's mind was sick with fear.

One night the young man had a dream... In his dreaming, he was awakening to the feeling of running like a wolf... but not just any wolf. This very special and unique Paq'tism was of Two Spirits, and had much to teach our young man...

Wanderer

We have taken journey through whole deserts. Climbed huge mountain chains. Walked through fire and burned off all my clothing. I have talked to strange and hidden entities in deep and dark forests. Walked for endless miles along meandering rivers of green... and stopped to hear the sound of feet that came over distant glens, and then, they called me back.

At whose voice I asked, 'Who goes there? Say your name if you will'. What I heard gave me pause. A lone wolf let out a harrowing cry and before me the moon, full and rising, came over the horizon just then, filling the stream with a pale-yellow hue, covering the trees about the edges of my consciousness with a vibrancy and expectation.

And I looked toward the sound of his cry. And saw stretching out before me a lengthening shadow unlike any I have ever seen before or since. It seemed to have a life all its own. It became detached from my solid form and danced toward the forest edge where shrubs guarded the way into a sacred grove. I hastened to walk toward its retreat into the wood, but fear gripped my bones until I fell headlong into the slippery earth lining the stream. I did fall, smashing my head on the rough-hewn stones. The last sound that I remember was the howl of the Paq'tism crying to the moon rising.

Waking Up

A short time later, I awoke and was bleeding still. The blood did not seem to clot, and when I inspected the wound in the clear reflection of the water, trickles of red fell into the still pool forming circles of expanding ringlets, never ending, reaching outward until the slow and steady current of the stream carried them away.

In my dizziness I felt my life flowing freely before my eyes, like the stream, and I became a dark black bird rising above the valley's edge, seeing everything expand, even peering thru these narrow but all-seeing eyes.

The beginnings were clear. As if far off, I could see where I began my journey twenty-eight years ago. The end of my time on this planet was just beyond my vision. But that which lay in between, I could remember and would yet walk… an ever-changing path of jagged corners around convoluted streams and high mountain ranges down steep and terrible precipices to lonely, uninhabited valleys and still, silent places. I remembered my shadow. The memory caused in me some alarm.

Rising Up on Wings

So, I looked toward the sacred grove where last I saw his retreat. Flying there, the trees passed beneath my wings. A mound of earthen design came into view. It lay in a semi-circle toward the moon, which was now at its zenith in the Southern sky. At its two arms the mound sloped toward the grassy earth, its highest point at its back where these arms met. Inside there was nothing save flat grassy earth, and how did I know? It was here where this world's realm meets and embraces all that is.

The grove was bright in the light of night's clarity. I flew toward the trees lining the grove and perched not far above, so that the great round moon was on my back, the circle's inner sanctuary was facing me.

We sat there for what seemed ages, all through the night, until the sky's darkness began to fade. The time between times was nearing. As the pale light of the Eastern sky began to shift and grow, I saw my wounded body break through the trees. There, inside the sacred mound, was my shadow, standing tall and defiant. Its voice bellowed like thunder, 'Stop where you stand!' My body froze in its tracks and trembled visibly, arms shaking at my sides.

Raven's Two Eyed Seeing

Perched like the Raven, I heard and watched … In a small frail voice, dried up. Parched.

Crisp was this voice, like the body which held so little blood, still laying on that stream's edge bleeding into the veins of mother earth. There came out of my bandaged head these tentative sounding words, 'I came to find you, you are mine. Why do you defy me?'

And my other form fell to her knees. Despair blanketed the grove like a heavy mantle. For long moments there was no sound, the air stood still to stop the sound of feet, the stream's distant voice receded until no life blood flowed in the world.

Everything became cold. Even the moon's strong light paled, grew dim, and a darkness covered the earth like hopelessness and cloud shadow.

Paq'tism Arising

From out of the thick mist, Paq'tism slowly peeked out. First a nose, smelling the damp air about this grove. Then one paw, then another... Stealth on graceful wings that touched mother earth with silent yet pulsing drums of power. But I did not see him. She of me looked from atop the tree, Raven's two eyed seeing. Her gaze penetrating.

From behind my huddled and weary form. Paq'tism crept close in stealth, and with his keen nose he sniffed the air for his game.

His legs were strong as Hemlock, his body hard as Oak, slick as Birch. His eyes shone forth in the darkness such that any creature who beheld their beauty would be transfixed, frozen as steel, and unable to resist being consumed by his beautiful and fierce teeth of silver, his warm breath like steam rising from hot mineral springs.

He crept up to my feet as I saw him from high above, he smelled and thought for a moment, what to do?

He backed off, as if to ward off danger. But he turned slightly, and walked around to my face, now with eyes closed as if in death.

Paq'tism licked my face and panted. I started. Frightened by my quick movement he ran a few feet away toward the sacred mound. And stood there, watching me. My form shifted, I looked into his eyes, and came back to myself.

Off, toward the Eastern sunrise, a Raven flew. I had only to know because I saw her shadow across the trees. And I thanked her silently for her gift of sight. Her being within me and my spirit was yet strange but comforting.

Paq'tism Awakening

Paq'tism's eyes held me fast, assessing me, looking as if into the pits of my very soul. How could I look away? Shame filled me like spit on my face. Like the boys that taunt me in school who beat my body, fallen to the ground. Like dying leaves of amber, reds, yellows, brown and black rosary beads hanging themselves by a lonely swimming pool. What Two Spirit might jump in never to surface again? We have died many deaths, like this, and many times…

This shame makes me want to vomit. But truth be told, after eons of shame, all there is left in me is this blood flowing from my wounds. Falling out of me into the stream. From empty heart to water of life… my purpose in all of this? Only sadness grips me.

Paq'tism lets out a harrowing cry. In his eyes another two eyed seeing came to light. I saw there the seething cauldron of inner transformation. How did he know? The demon hosts that danced and flew around its boiling, molten liquid, making grotesque acclamations, and feeding off each other's shame and fear? It came to me then, in Paq'tism's eyes. In the mirror of those wolverine eyes this cauldron of transformation awaited me. This was why I came here, into this skin-time. This is why the dreaming. The wandering. The loneliness all these years… This must surely be. A sacred ritual would now begin…

But wait. Grinding of other teeth. Resistance and futility. These demons drew back in horror at my realisation, seething and jeering at me, clawing and eating away the edges of my sanity. But even in my weakness and kindness of spirit I fought with them. I would not give in to their malice. But then so quickly we began to lose the fight that something in me snapped. The tension was too great!

I looked around, all was red and fire. I saw nothing. This so often happens and gives me shame. In the midst of any exchange, my racing mind and heart fails to see. The emotion and confusion in me. The feelings of other hearts outweigh me. Sensations not my own overwhelm and sustain this conflated sympathy. Your feelings make me crazy for loving, mad for quiet and peace. I was blind. Two eyed blindness. I was without sight.

When you feel so much, you sometimes freeze. But in this shameful silence of heartfelt noise, I heard the waters of the deep Birchbark cauldron speak to me an urgent word, 'We await the ritual of rebirthing, begin now, before it be too late'.

Surrender… Please…

We shifted again and assumed Indian sitting position. I let my bloody hands rest on my knees, open, in supplication. I knew this wolf was no stranger to me, and he held me still, in his wisdom and cunning.

A singular voice came from somewhere, at first, I thought it fell from storm clouds raising arms of war around the darkened moon.

Then we realised it came from a closer place, I forced my weary mind to hear. And like a rush of wind through sultry reeds beside the stream, I realised. It was my own throat that issued these words from some deep pit of darkness I never knew existed within me: 'Come close to me.'

And Sa'qawei Paq'tism walked closer, he knew the ritual which we were now beginning. This ritual was the reason why he was given to my protection as a child in the woods of Hatchet Lake, where I wandered in his lonely ways, seeking what was too great for me to grasp in those formative days.

The whole story of our lives together, of the intervening years of silence, the lone paths, the searching and darkness… it all came back to me then. It all came back to this one night of dark and frightening revelation.

This was the end for us. There would be no more of life or love, truth or beauty in this world's realm, for death is the cost of transformation. Every kernel of truth and irrelevancy would here be shed in the cauldron of Paq'tism's eyes.

As he drew close to me, I felt another shift of my body, but I stayed, resisting the urge to move.

An axe fell from somewhere high, fell fast and rang in my ears. It sank deep into my head but did not harm me, and I remembered in a flash - the hospital room where a nurse was sowing fourteen stitches in my bloody scalp.

And I remembered crawling on the ground toward the unfinished steps of the house in Hatchet Lake, 'Help me, I'm bleeding.'

And instantly I saw a five-hundred-year-old cut of cedar, standing upright, three feet high; its roots still pulling into the earth, round about. A green emerald handed axe was stuck in its centre, ringlets of hundreds of years expanded outward like ripples on the water.

Mother Earth groaned and heaved a sigh of pain. It was then I noticed that moist bubbling foam issued forth from the sides of the axe while the lifeblood of the ancient Spirit Tree was spilled out.

Shadow as Passage to Life

Coming back to myself, Paq'tism, drawing near me... Like we could reach out and soothe his neck and back, but my arms were like lava, heavy and flowing with a weird energy that fell as thickening blood from the tips of my fingers. I felt a wave of nausea begin to rise in my stomach and knew this ritual must begin very soon. My strength was waning dangerously, I was losing the sight, and could no longer see in clear lines.

His wolverine eyes were drawing back behind a grey distance. The moment was ripe. I opened my mouth. Inwardly I said, 'Come to me.' He came close. A breath issued forth from my mouth, my last breath in this world's realm. His lips touched mine, he accepted my offering. It was done.

Through his eyes my form slumped down, my head rested precarious on his face. I was dead. But I could still see through these eyes wide as ripe dandelions and clear as precious emeralds. He covered my mouth with his large jaw and pushed a breath like fire and ice deep into my lungs. Then he was gone. I fell sidelong, lying like a knot on the damp welcoming earth.

There was nothing more I could do. But my dreams rose up within to show me my defiant shadow sat huddled in a corner of the circled mound, her arms and feet severed. She could not move. She looked with horror at her appendages lying in front of her, torn and jagged, as if my friend the wolf had bitten them through, until they fell where they now lay, helpless.

But alas, my shadow was crying, tears of black like seams of liquid coal streamed down her cheeks and onto the grass. I never imagined a shadow could cry. Instinctively, I took these lifeless arms and legs into my hands, I was yet lying on my stomach, too weak to rise any higher. In my hands they rested and seemed to glow an eerie black light like the stone of hematite coming to life. Their heaviness shifted and evaporated until there was nothing left in my hands, there was only this sweaty residue making the veins in my palms look like massive crossroads and endless, untrodden ways.

A subtle strength came to me then, coming not from my heart or soul, but from the extremities of my being. As if my fingers and toes were sucking in a new life blood to replace that which was lost, as if the edges of my sanity were returning to me after a long sojourn in the desert of dreamless sleep. I felt the urge to rise, but this time I was actually able to do it in fact. I rose to my knees and knelt close to my crying shadow, still totally unaware of my presence.

Embracing Shadows

Deep, abiding pity filled me, and something like compassion chased away my fear. I no longer feared my shadow. I looked closer, could it be?

I strained my eyes to see, there, on the earthen mound, her tears seemed to disappear and reappear again. Where his tears fell on the grass of the sacred grove, I realised a slow germination was taking place. A transformation. A rebirth.

Before me there rose up little green things, from out of the grass, becoming taller, growing steady: But all the while, my shadow kept her crying vigil, unable to see, too introspective to hear the music of her own genesis.

The moon was black now behind a thick cloud covering, and rain was threatening to fall. But all that dared touch these green growing stems were her tears, and that was enough to confer on them the strength which looks through death.

But in her despair and terrible fear of discovery, my shadow remained powerless and dismembered. She continued to cry. The agony rose from her chest, choking her. I wanted to move to her, to help, to speak just one word. I lay there on the earth. We remained separate, confined in our prisons. I dead and they are dying. But she was all I had remaining. And yet, she couldn't see. And it was this not seeing which mattered more to me than anything. Something had to happen! How could we see as one being, whole and entire? How might those two eyes converge?

If only… To pierce the heart of the flower. To jump through that inner circle to that sacred land apart. Where deer come across my path in the early morning. They talk to me. They share the most ancient and sacred medicine.

Like when a child in the deep woods, waiting, silence, in reverence and awe. To reach into that heartfelt sacred place. To remain there for more than a millisecond. To pull back that medicine from the other realms, and touch and be touched within this sadness. This earth world of empty shadows. There is a music that sounds of Isness. There is a song of doves we can hear, even in despair.

Still, we couldn't. And we could not. But even then, we didn't notice. All around us time expanded. In spite of our spirit blindness small buds began to appear… There bloomed Roses crimson, and pale white Lilies among fragile purple Orchids.

Part of me could see but we were mostly blind. The sight of fear and despair living so close to the beautiful freedom of a garden of flowers confused me. It was too much for my flouting soul to bear.

Two Spirits Becoming Whole

We then felt the earth shake like the crushing of bone against bone. Wanting to jump and run, we were stuck in this rut of self-pity and shame. The very foundations of this world's realm shifted uncontrollably and would never be the same again. Surely our ancestors remember this fearful shaking of the worlds when all things begin anew. I awoke ever slowly.

The sun was just about to rise. Sunrise Ceremony? We realised that the time between times would end very abruptly and very soon, and my last chance to complete this ritual would pass forever.

We forced this weary body to crawl around. Oh, it seemed so slow. My every movement sent shards of pain shattering through my brain. Every nerve ending begged me to stop, to lie still, but I knew my time was short and the road to my recovery all too long.

Young Paq'tism'skw was only a few feet away, still Crying. Eyes so swollen from tears. Could not see my approach. Ears so plugged by this infection of sadness. Never heard my scraping body on the earth between us.

I reached out finally and touched that body's severed parts. They were cold as ice. Strange, I thought. My shadow should be warm. But then I realised, these appendages had been lying there for decades. Almost four long decades. Of course, they would be cold. Almost like stones in their abject condition. Tattooed with etchings of old colonial ships and long forgotten memories of medicine circles and ravens.

In one movement I lifted up my shadow with both arms in a singular and heartfelt embrace. We took the stubs of these arms and held her there, like long lost kin. We cried in joy.

She was now mine to hold, not to command, but to freely embrace. As a lover holds their beloved. She never realised what was happening, so deep and wounded this shadow remained. But I stayed there with her and waited.

How was it that the masculine was weaker than the feminine in the heart of our shadow? And even more sensitive was he to past trauma? Such is how the life of men's and women's sacred medicine unfolds. He may dance in the heart of the circle, but the woman carry the circle from around and about. They are the strong ones in spirit and heart. Their first medicine carries the nation in the time between times, and until this world's realm passes away. Was it centuries? Was it ten by ten by ten of years? I held on. And realised that I could never, never let go. Never again.

We stayed there, in the garden of flowers, and seasons came and went all around us. Skin times flew by like fast forwarded movies. Of trekking the ice shields, exploring the newly exposed tundra, then walking the deep forests.

Flouting upon the waves of time where loons came and went, still ready to raise their young. But in our sacred mound, time expanded to the break of day as one moment stretched to the edge of infinity.

Post-Trauma Recovery

This sorrow abated somewhat, only after what seemed many lives and deaths and cycles and seasons. But in spite of our rebirthing again and again, my sorrowful shadow never really disappeared.

In my age, in the time toward my ending days, I discovered these simple truths which have eluded me until now. In my need I found my source of wisdom. In my weakness was my strength. I had walked the pilgrim's way of solitude, sacrifice and service. But I had failed to abide my own frailty. I had failed to embrace my humanity. And in so doing, my life-quest had not yet begun.

It then came to me that sadness itself is a boon from Creator. Why and how could that be so? On the day of my awakening, I arose from the sacred mound and walked from the hallowed grove with the confidence of a Two Spirit who knew their totems.

From that time on my life unfolded as it should. I did not walk away alone however. Now with my befriended shadow, we walked together, mysteriously and silently. Shadow following me ever onward.

But truth be told, I listen more now. Listening to shadow's voice… Such inner wisdom this Two Spirit gives when least expected. She feeds the soul of me. We have never to fear her departure again. She is now part of me.

Sa'qawei Paq'tism Speaks

Like an Elder once said, there was at one time, back in the old days before internet and phones and all these gizmos, a rather young person. We lived on the edge of a great forest. Perhaps the very last forest to have existed. Who had suffered greatly with loss, grief, and anger.

This young Two Spirit felt inside the pull between anger and love. They had both violence and kindness welling up inside of them.

The war was so strong this young one's mind was soul sick with fear. Maybe this was why they could not accept Two Spirit nature that over the years starts welling up inside the body?

Sometimes all we need to do is breathe… like this… take your air inside of you. Yes… sacred air from the World Above the Earth. Sacred… Hold it inside. And then release…

This circle goes on like a spiral sea shell all our days, as long as this skin-time continues. We carry this Medicine. But you see, this powerful Two Spirit Way is both sadness and joy. Both anger and kindness. Both this way and that way. To dance with your own wolves, you need to dance with your inner shadows too.

So yes, as you now know, one very special night when the stars were all shiny and bright, and the moon was going full and wild, our young one had a dream…

In sacred dreaming, there was an awakening to the feeling of running like a wolf… but not just any wolf… This very special and unique Paq'tism was of Two Spirits with much to teach our young Mi'kmaq…

When all was said and done, our youthful old soul once again walked out of that sacred mound transformed in reconciliation. The anger was gone but could come back. Anger is like this. When we harness the energy, we learn to channel that same energy. This is a skin-time skill you practice over the moons. Power rises. Power falls. And power always exists in nature. This is the way of things.

But I wonder somehow if our young Two Spirit Puoinaq ever really left that sacred grove. If perhaps the rest of that skin-time was a memory or vision from that place where they first embraced. Yes, it is true at least, that life in the land of the living begins on that night's end when the day has not yet begun. And to Paq'tism, these words we now transcribe, in memory of Two Spirit wisdom and breath of rebirth, 'Never fear the embrace of your shadows, they are not as fearsome as at first they may appear.'

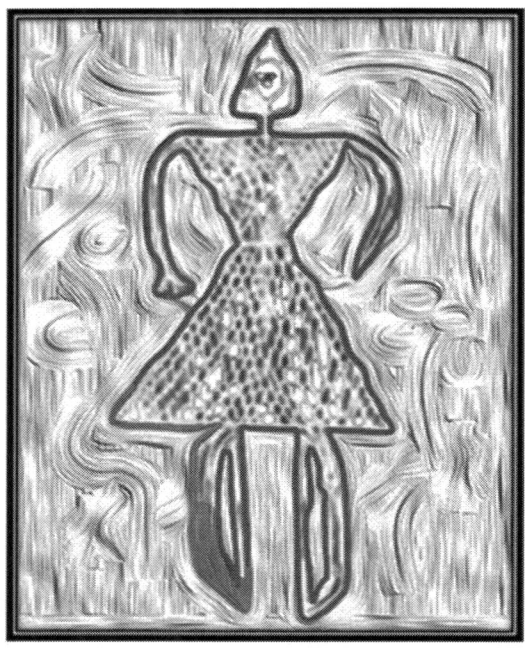

'Through the Dreaming and the Medicine, we vision and journey. The sound of the Drum carries us across the worlds. The Drum Beat carries us to the Heart of Creation.'

Two Spirit Narrative of Origins

Pjila'si, welcome, come in, sit down. Welcome again to our sacred fire. Come closer, stay warm. Kwe, greetings from the Eastern Door of Turtle Island.

We wish you to imagine a time long ago, when a very old Elder of the people sat by the fire of her Wigwam. She burned sage to purify the body and the air around about. Calling in the directions, listening, and staring into the fire.

Your place was by the Wigwam door. You waited in silence for the right time to make your offering. When it was time, the Elder looked into your corner and waited to meet your eyes.

You offered the Ancient One gifts of Sacred Tobacco that you had spent a great deal of time to find and money to trade. You gave gifts of practical food, and items the Elder could use in daily life. You knew that their work prevented them from keeping a regular job. As healer and teacher and seer, their path was different. So, you gave to them with generous heart, because you asked great things of them.

When the gifts were accepted, the Old One said, 'What do you seek?' You asked, 'Please share with me the story of our origins. We wish to know the Two Spirit Way.'

Taking up Sacred Turtle Rattle, the Most Ancient of Medicines, the Old One of the People leaned into the fire. Stoking the coals with a stick. Putting more Sage upon the coals. She began to chant an Ancient Melody.

Taking Sweet Grass, the Elder Puoinaq leaned closer into the fire. Raising that Sweet Grass high into the air, burning the Sacred Herb of the Ancestors, your mind began to still and sway, as if beginning to swim in the organic sounds of voice and rhythmic patterns of the Grandmother's Turtle Rattle. It was as if you heard these words of the Kji'puoinaq'skw echoing through the years…

Kepmitelsi Two Spirit Pride

'We honour the North Eastern woodlands of the continent of North America. With our families and elders, we say M'sit No'kama, All My Relations. This saying conveys the sacred ways of our People and our Spiritual Beliefs. We are all one in creation. And each one has a special place, a purpose, and a calling, given by Creator.

'We come from a tradition that honours the soul or spirit of each person regardless what they are made of or who they come to be. In our way, we honour diversity because we see and experience this diversity in all of creation around us – our Sacred Land and Water is rich with great diversity and plenty.

'Why would we ever discount or put aside any part of this wonderful and beautiful creation? To do so would dishonour the Creator. To do so would be to commit harm upon that which is perfect, not because we wish anything to be perfect, but because we acknowledge that the way things are in creation is given to us to teach us valuable lessons – we do not mess with creation.

'We respect the nature around us and within us, in our family, and in our nation. We are all kin and have special relations of power, knowledge, and communication with Spirits from Animal, Bird, Plant, Water, Stone and Star nations. These many Peoples we respect. Some are given to us personally, in our family, and for our nation, for special purposes. We listen to that wisdom, and the teachings that come with these good relations.

'Within a familial and community ethic of respect and honour we remember that the Two Spirit being came about during the very first days of creation, long before the days of the Old Ones of the People. This is why their spirits are called 'Sa'qawei,' or Ancient…

'Those were the times when the Stone and Water nations were arguing over the boundaries of Land and Sea. Those were the times when the Mountain Nations were first being formed on this Grand Island of the Sacred Turtle Elders. Spawned from the ancient seed of the Elder Turtle Nation the Two Spirit Puoinaq first came into being. This was a time of great upheaval and uncertainty when the tides of existence were held in the balance.

'Huge seismic eruptions were causing enormous changes throughout the Earth World. All the six and eight Sacred Worlds were caught within the first drama of creation, because creation itself includes the powers of destruction and these together are part of this sacred mystery we call transformation.

'Such was the drastic differences from later times. Even the Forest and Tree Nations were not yet in existence! It was during this expansive time of tremendous conflicts and arguments between the Stone Nation and the Water Nation that the Two Spirit beings came together in Sacred Council.

Ancient Old Ones - Two Spirit Beings

'Knowing how much pain was being caused by petty arguments and misunderstandings, and being naturally drawn to balance, beauty, and harmony, with playful and passionate feelings, the Ancient Old Ones, the Two Spirit Elders met in Council and in private, as they are wanting to do when they discuss the hidden secrets of the nations. Over many days and nights of fasting and prayer by the Sacred Fire of the Turtle Elders they together decided that enough was enough.

'The Puoinaq spoke as one voice and said that the Stone and Water nations had to face their differences. Something must come from their reconciliation, after all, they had been eyeing each other off for thousands of moons without any result whatsoever. As you might guess, nothing drove the Ancient Two Spirits more into madness and crazy mind than seeing people argue who could be making love.

'In an unprecedented move, the Oldest Among Them leaned forward, raised an arm to silence the group, and stood up Tall and Strong. Others slowly rose to their feet and waited, until everyone was standing around the Sacred Fire of the Council Wigwam of the Ancient Two Spirit Elders. It was then that the Oldest Among Them shared their heart, moving that the Ancient Magic of the Spheres was needed to save Turtle Island from disaster, which was surely to happen if this madness was not stopped and forgiveness for the past hurts between the nations was not healed once and for all time.

Conference of the Four Winds

'In the moons that followed, a call went out across the land and sea from The Puoinaq Council. The message was clear. It was to be set in time a Grand Council of the Four Winds to be hosted by the Eastern Door of Turtle Island. This was long before the Mi'kmaq Nation came to be born, but that part of the story comes later. No one except the Two Spirit Elders in their Secret Council knew the real purpose of this Inaugural Conference of Nations. Even the Stone Nation and the Water Nation had no idea of what was to come.

'During the Summer Moon, the Loon Nation was called to prepare the feast, and showing their generosity of spirit and awesome hospitality the Finned Ones offered of their own accord to give of their lives so that the members of the Sacred Council would have good and excellent feed upon their long and difficult journey across the face of Mother Earth.

'The time drew near for the Conference of the Grand Council of the Four Winds. Mother Earth herself set the Sacred Fire that would burn for Seven Moons before the High Tide that struck the beginning of the Grand Council of the Four Winds. During these moons the Ancient Two Spirits fasted and prayed, sacrificed, and sought visions from across the Sacred Worlds of Creation.

'These were the days long before the Old Ones of the People, and after the revealing of a very special Dream, the Two Spirit Elders determined that an exceptional measure was needed to host and entertain the Visitors from the Four Winds. It came about one day when a vision came to one of the younger Two Spirits.

The Two Spirit Vision

'She came to her sisters and said, 'I saw a very long, I mean a really long wigwam in my dreams. It looked so strange! But inside, all the Sacred Visitors were seated around a huge warm fire, and the walls were decorated with sacred designs from the twigs and herbs brought in by the Tree and Herb Nations. It smelled so lovely! At either end was an entrance, and in the other sides a passage way, so there was a flow of energy from the Four Winds throughout the wigwam.'

'Those that heard the Sacred Dream began to weep. Their hearts were so touched that their knees went weak, as often happens with Two Spirits, and they nearly fell to the ground weeping with tears of joy and happiness. In that moment they realized in their hearts that the Dream was a foretelling of a time of richness and plenty, when the children of the nations would be at peace and sharing their lives in harmony and balance – and this they saw was the exact fulfilment of the Two Spirit purpose given by the Creator for all nations. Their hearts were filled with great courage and strength in their purpose.

'After that day, with great sanctity there was prepared the first ever Long House, which was decorated with very special seven-pointed designs made from whatever gifts creation had to offer at that time. Remember, the forests had not yet grown, the land was in a big mess, so the Two Spirits did what they do best, and they made beautiful and lovely what was ugly and boring. They used painted stone, woven grasses, seashells beaded in wonderful sparkling designs with woven seaweed forming large wall adornments, and many other natural elements drawn together for the occasion. It was for no small purpose that the Long House was made ready as if for a wedding feast of nations. By the time they had finished, the Long House was fit for the finest of Chiefs and Dignitaries from the Four Winds.

'Even during the early days nearing this Sacred Council the Two Spirit Elders heard of enormous battles between the Stone Nation and the Water Nation. It seemed to them that they truly wished to destroy all hope for Turtle Island, and to crush any chances of survival for all the nations of Mother Earth. The turmoil was so great and to such a degree that the land Herself shuttered with the fierce anger of war. Mountains were appearing where there had been none.

'Lakes were completely drained and became barren, and rivers changed their course overnight, while eruptions of fluids, gasses, and ash changed the landscape and caused great discontent among the nations. The Land kept expanding as if she wanted to dominate and control the whole surface of Mother Earth, pushing with violent rage and anger toward the Water nation.

'The Water nation on her part made the oceans themselves rise up with fierce anger and washed upon the land destroying everything in sight, moving and churning, again and again, as if wanting to claim the whole earth for herself and knowing that she of all nations held the most power and would win this war in the end.

Ancient Grandmother Turtle Pipe

'But as was known and agreed by Ancient Law, upon the Opening of the Sacred Sunrise Ceremony of the Two Spirit Elders in the Eastern Door, where Grandfather Sun first touches the Eastern most point of Turtle

Island, the war between the Stone and Water Nations must cease during the Seven Sacred Days of the Grand Council of the Four Winds.

'During the Opening Ceremony, the oldest and most respected Two Spirit Medicine Keeper raised the Most Ancient Turtle Nation Pipe. Unlike all pipes that have come and gone, this first pipe drew together the powers of Stone, Air, Water, and Fire into one being in the body of the first Turtle. This pipe bowl carried the most Ancient Water for healing and blessing of body.

'The Sacred Water was taken through a beautifully carved stone stem to the lips of the Two Spirit Elder. Coming from the First Primal Medicine Dreaming this Sacred Grandmother's Turtle Pipe drew in all the Old Magic of Earth, Sea, Wind, and Flame. No one would dare whisper a word in the presence of this Sacred Elder.

'All were silent. In the distance outside the Inner Circle Water Nation stood, watching and waiting. Closer to the circle Stone Nation had come to listen to what was said, curious what the Two Spirit would say. To great surprise, without delay and with dramatic effect, the Elder carried the Nation Pipe to the Centre of the Circle and stood over the Sacred Fire, raised their head to the Sky Nation, and prayed a Prayer of Forgiveness.

'As they prayed their body rose above the Sacred Fire, and those who looked on saw in the flames of time the Many Faces of the Nations come forward. Nations that were not yet in existence, dreamed up by the Elder Puoinaq. Among these faces in blended mirage were the Nations of the Wolf, Bear, Eagle, Humming Bird, Otter, Beaver, Moose, Lynx, and Porcupine. Among these faces arose the White Buffalo Calf and the Albino Moose Women who eons later dreamed again the Teachings of the Sacred Pipe lost for so long among the ancient tides of this mysterious planet.

'Each person around the Gathering were transfixed and listened with gaping open mouths to every word. Those that needed translation were offered by the Ones with Gifted Tongues. During the Prayer and while the Nation Pipe was lifted high above the Sacred Fire, everyone felt nearly compelled to come closer, closer, and still closer as the Two Spirit Elder whispered the most precious and delicate prayer that melted every heart and moved everyone to tears.

'As they were so drawn into the Sacred Energy of that Prayer of Forgiveness, their hearts melted away. When the prayer was nearly finished, those gathered there felt as if they were opening their eyes for the first time... Around the Fire stood Stone Nation on the Western Door and Water Nation on the Eastern Door. No one noticed at first, but there was a subtle energy that had shifted. The Great Power of that Two Spirit Elder was manifested without anyone realizing, and only the other Old Two Spirits knew. They quietly made eye contact with each other, as they often do without anyone else realizing their communication.

'Silently, during the Council, magic was happening all around the People of the Four Winds. Meals of wonderful fish, and herbs, and salads from the land appeared whenever they were needed. The Two Spirits signalled to each other the needs of various dignitaries and saw that their wishes were fulfilled before they even whispered their thoughts between their two ears. Such was the amazing contentment and peace of that Inaugural Conference that one day it was found quite without notice that two Nations were standing alone by the Sacred Fire, both were offering Sage and Tobacco to the Flames of the Mother, one standing in the East, the other in the West.

Two Spirit Healing of Nations

'They looked into each other's eyes, as if for the first time. They gazed at each other with a naked understanding. From within their bodies arose a spontaneous longing that they had never before known or realized. How strange, they each thought, what magic is possessing me? But they were compelled to each other with a simple but irresistible desire.

'This was just enough for them to bridge the distance between them, as they resisted coming closer together. But the pull was too strong. For the first time they saw an accord to live together in relationship and in peace. It was then, in that very moment, that silence fell over Turtle Island. All of mother earth became still... like the water of Black Rattle Lake upon a clear early morning, when the mist hovers gentle over a crystal glass expanse.

'From that time on, it was known that Stone Nation became joined with Water Nation in Sacred Union, and from their consummation during a much later time arose the Sacred Dawn of Glooscap son of Creator whose tides of awakening brought about the time of the children of Men and children of Women. This was how the creation song brought about such young spirits who had never lived before on Turtle Island.

'From these youthful spirits and during a much later time the Mi'kmaq Nation sprang up like weeds on a sunny and warm day in July. After that time, the Nation of Two Legged was formed of the diversity of Men Spirits and Women Spirits, who spawned many babies that needed much caring, nurturing and protection from harm. As you might guess, much like your mom and dad, these Men and Women spirits were young and immature. They did not know how to be parents. They did not even know how to care for themselves!

Teaching the First Mi'kmaq

'So much more like the ancient Stone and Water Nations at war, these new Mi'kmaq men and women were very much prone to arguing against each other and among themselves. They had much to learn. They did not know how to live, let alone, how to live in peace and harmony. They did not even have passion and love, because they had not learned those lessons during those days. Raising their own children was an even larger task that they failed to do with any certainty or skill. After all, they could hardly even take care of themselves.

'Over many, many moons the People with Two Legs began to revere the Two Spirit Old Ones who actively taught them the lessons and skills they needed to live in harmony and peace. It was during these times that the People created songs and dances and remembered these through their Sacred Song Lines. In music it was taught about how to love, how to forgive, and how to raise children with kindness, respect, and gentleness. Over eons of time added to these primal ways of the People were teachings about how to hold the Sacred Medicine Pipe, and how to skilfully craft family and personal Pipes to keep the Sacred Flame of Forgiveness alive in the many moons that followed.

'The Two Spirit Old Ones during this time worked in concert with the Old Ones of the People, our Ancestors. They helped the People care for their children. They tended fire. They cooked while the women were on their moon time. They crafted useful tools from wood and stone. They hunted game in the forest. They became known among the People during these days as the greatest craftsmen, storytellers, and Keepers of the Medicine and Dreaming.

'The Two Spirit Old Ones held the memory of who could marry who, so they also kept the People strong and healthy. They held the spiritual knowledge of all the many plants that came to grow with their help and inspiration. Their spiritual power worked with the Creator during the times when new species were being formed to assist the People in their wellbeing. These were the days of the Two Spirit Medicine Keepers that seemed to last for endless moons.

Prophesies of the Great Suffering

'During those days of living in peace and harmony among the Old Ones of the People, and during the time of the Long House when the People lived in the abundance of the land and sea, the Two Spirit Medicine Keepers foresaw that their time of direct custodianship of the Sacred Worlds would draw to an end. During those days they gathered together from across the Mi'kmaq nation to meet again in Secret Two Spirit Council.

'Deliberating what to do, they fasted and prayed once again during a cycle of seven sacred moons. It was then that a deep sorrow and grief for what was to come arose within the Two Spirit Medicine Keepers as they foresaw a future time of great upheaval, death, disease, domination and fear. In their visions came the near extinction of the People from the face of Mother Earth. Within their spiritual beings they gave up their power in prayer and sacrifice to prevent that extinction and turn the tides of power for the sake of the nation and the families they had come to love and serve.

'As the seven sacred moons came to a close, during the time of the Spring Solstice, the Puoinaq Council met again in the quiet reach of the forest where silence and peace was most profoundly felt, and where the spirits of creation could be consulted without distraction. They determined in Council that on one hand their spiritual power would always be needed among the People.

'But on the other hand, they had to acknowledge that a time of great suffering was coming unlike anything the People had endured up to that time. The most sensitive among them saw that this time of darkness and death would come to be such that even their spiritual power would not be welcomed among the People. Due to the great pressures and catastrophes that would befall the nation, even the Two Spirit would be cast out by their own families. While this greatly disturbed the Two Spirit, they also were wise enough to know that something needed to be done.

'To carry the memory of their power deep in the heart of the People, during that Spring Ceremony so many moons ago, the Two Spirit Medicine Keepers planted the seed of exceptional giftedness within the joining of the spirits of Stone Nation and Water Nation. This spiritual seed multiplied the fruitfulness of the joining through the addition of passion and love. With passion and love men and women spirits began to fall in love, fire and air. This was how the first nation pipes entered the Dreaming. This was well before the days of the White Buffalo Calf and Albino Moose Women. and share a fullness of compassion, understanding, and a greater potential for acts of kindness.

The First Two Spirit Mi'kmaq

'During that Spring Ceremony the Two Spirit Old Ones gave the nation an equally important gift. They extended their spiritual power to fusing the spirits of the Stone and Water nations in such a way that from time to time, and in an unpredictable manner, the Ancient Two Spirits would be reborn within the families of the nation. Without reason or warning they would be born within chosen families as a gifted presence hidden and secret until such time that the ancient spirit medicine awakens in that child later in life. This was how it came to be that someone could live out their lives in the body of a Two Legged being while always knowing they are somehow different, in some ways very unique.

'This was how it came to be that the first Two Spirit Elders were born into the bloodlines of the families of the Mi'kmaq nation. This was how the Two Spirit came to walk between the worlds of Men and Woman and to carry the Medicine and Dreaming of both Stone and Water Nations within their one body. This is why many very astute elders within the nation today see how the Two Spirit are called to model for the People in their very being a spiritual presence and a way of living in harmony, balance, and beauty, because they see within us this giftedness of both Stone Nation and Water Nation spirits.

'During the latter days of the Long House it was then that within the heart of the nation arose deeper power of resilience and courage. The gifts of the Two Spirit Old Ones tapped into the very energy of hope from the Heart of Mother Earth that rose up within each person to allow them to sacrifice their own personal needs for the needs of others. These were the days when the teaching on hospitality came to be so important for the nation. These were the times of great feasts and entertainment, fun and enjoyment, when the nations gathered together under the Confederacies of the Sacred Pipe.

'And this gave rise to that period of time we know as the days of the Talking Stick Circle and the Sweat Lodge Ceremony. These were the days of great purification. Even though many of our People were not aware, these days gave the People the very power they needed to survive the longest winter of sorrows that was to come. By the time the young woman saw the vision of the flouting islands from across the great waters, the Two Spirit Elders ancient visions had come to pass. Change was now upon us.

'It was then that the People sent Two Spirit Medicine Keepers. They sent them to greet the white skin who came down from the flouting islands. Our Two Spirit Ancestors took the role of ambassador during the first encounters with the Europeans.

'How strange it must have been for the white skin to see from their own eyes their projection of a gender deviant male of great physical prowess and beauty, confidence and grace, dressed in the style of the day with long flowing hair, feathers, and many decorations of carved bone, quill, shell, and seed. No wonder from their limited view they saw only a savage, a male gone wild, with none of the self-constraints, limitations, and cultural taboos of their upbringing.

The Great Suffering

'The white skin viewed our family relations with distain. Unlike them we valued most of all our elders, our women and our children. The role of men was during those days to serve and protect, not to lord over or supervise and demand service from others. Men lived by example. Men showed their emotion freely and valued tenderness and allowed their weakness to be known by those around them. This was their greatest strength shown in honesty, openness, and honouring their own feeling so as to honour their loved ones and community with a willingness to listen, to change, and to grow as a person. Men spirits had, after all, first learned how to love and to be sensitive spirits from the most gifted Two Spirit Elders that walked among the Old Ones of the People.

'But over time things were corrupted and values corroded, to the point where the People lived in Great Confusion. These were the days of the Longest Winter that we foresaw so long ago when our People may not survive the genocide and extinction set upon us from the forces of other nations who desired with greed to take our land and sea, and to possess even our sacred teachings, as if they could presume to control and dominate the Stone and Water, Fire and Air nations from whom our People are given their spiritual life and human form.

'The Longest Suffering was endured through the sacrifices of so many of our Ancestors, including those Two Spirit Old Ones who give up their spiritual power time and again by being born into the families of the nation. Even when they face such great misunderstanding, and they feel so terribly alone, and the weight of suffering of the People is so extensive, still they come to our people.

'Yes, very sad. How some Two Spirit beings come to us as babies in the womb, and for some reason they cannot stay among us for very long… These young Two Spirits may in their way sacrifice themselves and release themselves from the pressures of the violence and harm that is happening even now among the People…

'In the World Above the Sky we know, we see how these Angels of Mercy come to help our families and nation. Never doubt the power of the Spirit given as gift to our families. Some Spirits are Twice Over, because they carry

Two not One. These gifted Ones are of the Medicine even when they are not awake.

A World for our Children

'We know we are called to change and to create a world where our children and youth no longer feel sorrow, shame, or violence. This has been the same for eons. Our times are special now, for we pray for the Old Ones but pray more for the Seventh Generation who will come in time… Their world will be in need of our Medicine, even more.

'We must awaken to the reality that Two Spirit beings wish to come into our families. Can you hear them? They are singing to you now. Listen to their song! They rest just outside of the birthing chambers of the Great Hall, that Wigwam of the Old Ones. Where Spirits are ordained to serve, to give their lives for others. That Chamber of Ancients where all nations come in humility and service. They come to help Male and Female spirits to awaken to parts of themselves that are more tender, more open, healthy, balanced, to become even stronger and more resilient.

'We need to remember that the greatest teachings arise from places of silence, spontaneous creativity, intuition and vision, giftedness and sensitivity, subtleness and beauty, balance and harmony. Yes… these are the spaces that the Two Spirit Nation live and breathe and make their Presence known among the youthful Mi'kmaq Nation.

'We must also realize how easy it is to upset this balance. Burn Sage and Juniper now… Raise the Sacred Pipes and bring in the Sacred Tobacco. It is time to honour the Ancient Two Spirit Old Ones of the People.

Visions of Hope

'To right the balance we journey into the future. In those times of the White Albino Moose there will arise Rainbows of Light upon the Morning. There will come feminine powers that have been sleeping for very long, since the time before times. Even the strongest of men will be shaken. And new pathways will emerge from the ashes.

'Be that we may give our babies a place of safety and loving kindness. Yet every loss must of course teach us. But how harsh the lessons when Two Spirit babies and young children encounter abuse and neglect. This is not our way. They like most children internalize the harm and become depressed and live within a trauma story.

'The sadness of this story is all they know for a long time… This has always been the case, even in the Old Ones and among their kin. Healing takes special medicine, but this healing is very possible. Indeed, healing can happen in the blink of an eye or the time it takes to sleep and rest. Our bodies hold enormous and ancient wisdom.

'But how slow healing can seem because adults who are so confused in their own trauma histories do not have the skills or abilities to nurture, to love, to support, and to open healing ways. We need to learn to open space for our infants and children to learn the pathways of self-acceptance, tolerance, patience, forgiveness, peace-making, and creativity of being.

'Two Spirits are given to us to teach. But first we need to help these gifted souls to grow up, to become the people our nation most needs. First Men and Woman spirits must grow strong enough inwardly to care for and protect their Two Spirit children. If we can do this, we will reap the rewards of a lifetime of surprising joy and fun as the Two Spirit grows into their being in fullness.

'We all need to know that we have a place within our families and in our nation. We need to know the story of our place and this story brings health and wellness through an identity of place, an identity of culture.

'Parents of Two Spirit children need to share these stories in pride of place. Then all children regardless what their ways, or how their unique body speaks and sings, or in what colourful ways their gender gives rise to expression or to sexuality and love making in respect and honour, then all these diversities might manifest freely, and we can feel at ease, welcomed, and embraced as part of the family. This is our dream for the future, for the Seventh generation.'

Healing and Recovery

You did not even realise, but all of a sudden the narrative was finished and the still beating Turtle Rattle was quickly shaken for a long while, as if to say, 'Ta'ho! It is Done!' Your eyes slowly focused again, for you had been lost in the flames of the Sacred Fire. And the Sweet Grass lingered in the air.

Your eyes fell upon the Old One leaning into her side. They looked ancient and very tired. Tears had been falling from their face, and somehow their skin looked burned and older than you had noticed before. As the energy of the Puoinaq Elder waned your heart sank even more so, as you pondered in the sacred silence the meanings of her Medicine Story. You wondered how she came to such wisdom. And you were grateful that magic was still existing, at least somewhere, to have brought this moment to light is surely a gift.

It is important to realize that this narrative arises out of enormous challenges and during a time when the native community is suffering the mourning and loss of youth from suicide, and when in primary ways the identity of members of the community is fractured due to trans-generational trauma, violence, sexual abuse, substance abuse, and post-traumatic stress. It is equally important to know that this story of our origins comes to light at this time of cultural and spiritual renewal when the traditions of the People are being rekindled, and the Sacred Fires reset.

To give voice to a narrative of Two Spirit healing and restoration is an important task. This is only a small and humble beginning. Yet the fragments are here. From this work you can rekindle the sacred fires of ancient and contemporary Two Spirit pathways.

As Two Spirit people we know that only when the least respected of our People are brought back into a Sacred Role with respect and honour, only then will the People seek healing. We understand that for whatever reasons the Two Spirit represent for the Mi'kmaw Elders a pathway to balance and beauty, harmony and maturity in spirit. Perhaps the Elders feel that when the least respected are brought back into the story with honour and respect, then all members of the community will also find a place. Perhaps also the blending in maturity and spiritual power of Male and Female spirits in one body represents a spiritual calling that the Elders feel is innate to all beings of light. This is somehow in our future and is the destiny of the Two Spirit being and of humanity as a whole. At once both ancient and contemporary, very much now and yet futuristic.

Two Spirit exists on that plane of being where only the Seventh Generation abides, in the space of the White Albino Moose Woman and the Sacred Medicine Pipe Carrier. Just the other day an image of the Sacred Moose came across my gaze. Much like the sacredness of the Buffalo, for we Mi'kmaq the Moose holds similar mystique and power. The animal harkens back to the ancient times of the last great winter. The living connection to the past is deeply felt by our people.

The Albino Moose is surely just as sacred and rare a creature as the plains Indian equivalent. In similar fashion, the deeply Mi'kmaw ways of Two Spirit teachings need to be reawakened and rekindled along our own pathways. Spirits of Moose, Deer, Lynx, Wolf, Eagle, Octopus, Salmon, Trout, Turtle, and many other Spirits of the Eastern Door and Fires of Sunrise will certainly help us on this journey.

In so many ways, the work ahead belongs to the younger elders whose lives are just beginning. This book is written for you who seek the old ways. But know full well that you need to live them in the modern and future worlds coming to be, even as you sleep. This wisdom will come to you. What you need will be there for you, even when you least expect this to happen…

There will be times when everything seems wrong. Even evil might be an apt word to describe the happenings all around you. The darkness and loss may seem overwhelming. You may even want to give up and leave this earth.

In these times, just know that Life is more than what you see and feel. Life with a Capital 'L' kind of way is the power of Creator who is actually still creating. If you ever made pancakes you know that getting the mix right takes a lot of wrist action! It is very messy! It does not come easily! How much more do you need to give Creator some slack for creating your life, your being, your Spirit?!

It may be messy at times, but one thing is for sure. Creator loves you beyond compare. You are 100% unique in this world. Yeah you may have been around the Circle of Life more than once, you might even be one of the Old Souls who has lived hundreds of thousands of skin-times. But the reality is that every person has to go through it all again… Shitty diapers! Colds and flu! Upset love affairs! Broken promises! Feeling alone, and lonely, and isolated!

All these things are part of being human at one time or other. And part of learning the Sacred Paths of Being. Sometimes we endure great darkness and cannot figure why because there is actually a much bigger picture. We can't see that now. We just do not have all the pieces. But they are all there, in potential, and Creator is sorting things out even while we sleep.

Our suffering is like how the Sweat Lodge teaches that there is a purpose, a reason, even when we cannot see. After all you cannot see in the darkness of the Sweat. This is a hard lesson to learn when you grow up with a mobile or cell phone. The Sweat Lodge may seem like a very scary place. Life is like this too at times.

After all, we don't need to see or feel to know that Life is all around us. Knowing is beyond feeling. Beyond thinking.

Life is a great Mother. When even our earthly mother fails and rejects us, there is still the Great Grandmother of Life. Even when our grandmothers are all gone, even then their Spirit lives on in our lives. She is in the rising of the sun. We see her in the ways the trees offer shade. We feel her on a rainy day, giving life to the earth. She will not let us fall. She will lift you up on Eagle's wings.

May your Medicine Dreamtime awaken you to new possibilities and always give you healing and strength.

Bibliography

Adams G., Fryberg S., Garcia D. and Delgado-Torres E. (2006) The psychology of engagement with Indigenous identities: A cultural perspective, Cultural Diversity and Ethnic Minority Psychology, 12(3), 493-508.

Anguksuar-LaFortune, R. (1997) A postcolonial perspective on western misconceptions of the cosmos and the restoration of indigenous taxonomies, In Jacobs, S., Thomas, W., and Lang, S. (Eds.) Two-spirit people: Native American gender identity, sexuality and spirituality, University of Illinois Press, Chicago, 217-222.

Appleby G. and Anastas J. (1998) Not just a passing phase: Social work with gay, lesbian, and bisexual people, Columbia University Press, New York.

Arguello T., Walters K. (2017) They tell us 'we don't belong in the world and we shouldn't take up a place': HIV discourse within two-spirit communities, Journal of Ethnic and Cultural Diversity in Social Work, http://dx.doi.org/10.1080/15313204.2017.1362616.

Arredondo P. (1999) Multicultural counselling competencies as tools to address oppression and racism, Journal of Counseling and Development, (78) Winter, 102-108.

Arthur N. and Collins S. (2010) Culture-Infused Counselling: Celebrating the Canadian Mosaic, Counselling Concepts, Calgary.

Atkinson J., Kennedy D., Bowers R. (2006) Aboriginal and First Nations approaches to counselling, In Pelling N, Bowers R., and Armstrong P. (Eds.), (2006) The practice of counselling, Thomson Publishers, Melbourne.

Balsam K., Huang B., Fieland K., Simoni J. and Walters K. (2004) Culture, trauma, and wellness: A comparison of heterosexual and lesbian, gay, bisexual, and Two Spirit Native Americans, Cultural diversity and ethnic minority psychology, 10(3), 287-301.

Battiste M. (2004) Animating sites of postcolonial education: Indigenous knowledge and the humanities, Paper presented at the CCSE Plenary Address, May 29, 2004, Manitoba.

Battiste M., Bell L., Findlay L. (2002) Decolonizing education in Canadian universities: An interdisciplinary, international, Indigenous research project, Canadian Journal of Native Education, 26(2), 82-95.

Battiste M., Bell L., Findlay L. (2002a) An interview with Linda Tuhiwai Te Rina Smith, Canadian Journal of Native Education, 26(2), 169-185.

Battiste M. (1998) Enabling the autumn seed: Toward a decolonized approach to Aboriginal knowledge, language, and education, Canadian Journal of Native Education, 22(1), 16-28.

Battiste M. (1977) Cultural transmission and survival in contemporary Mi'kmaq society, The Indian Historian, 10(4), 2-33.

Bishop, R. (2005) Freeing ourselves from neo-colonial domination in research: A Kaupapa Maori approach to creating knowledge, In Denzin, N. and Lincoln, Y. (Eds.), The SAGE handbook of qualitative research, 3rd Edition, Sage, Thousand Oaks, 109-138.

Blackwood, E. (1997) Native American genders and sexualities: Beyond anthropological models and misrepresentations, In Jacobs, S., Thomas, W., and Lang, S. (Eds.) Two-spirit people: Native American gender identity, sexuality and spirituality, University of Illinois Press, Chigago, 284-294.

Bockting, W., Kundson, G., and Goldberg, J. (2007) Counseling and mental health care for transgender adults and loved ones, In Bockting, W., and Goldberg, J. Guidelines for transgender care, Haworth Medical Press, NY, 35-82.

Bodi M. (2009) Stories for the past, present and future: Canadian colonialism and the emergence of Two-spirituality, Kanata, Undergraduate journal of the Indigenous studies community of McGill, McGill University, Vol. 2, 121-131.

Bowers R. (2013) On the threshold: Personal transformation and spiritual awakening – A primer on the spiritual life with activities, Earth Rattle Publishing, Armidale.

Bowers R. (2013) Sacred teachings from the medicine lodge, Earth Rattle Publishing, Armidale.

Bowers R. (2012) From little things big things grow, from big things little things manifest: An Indigenous human ecology discussing issues of conflict, peace, and relational sustainability, *AlterNative – International Journal of Indigenous Studies*, 8(3) 290-304.

Bowers R. (2011) Mapping competencies for entry to the counselling psychotherapy profession in Australia, *Counselling Australia*, 11(3), Spring, 4-16.

Jha, C., Plummer, D. Bowers, R. (2011) Coping with HIV and dealing with the threat of impending death in Nepal, *Mortality,16(1), 20-34.*

Bowers R. (2010) Identity, prejudice, and healing in Aboriginal circles: Models of identity, embodiment, and ecology of place as traditional medicine for education and counselling – A Mi'kmaq First Nation perspective, AlterNative – International Journal of Indigenous Studies, 6(3), 203-221.

Bowers R. (2010a) A Mi'kmaq First Nation cosmology: Investigating the practice of contemporary Aboriginal Traditional Medicine in dialogue with counselling – Toward an Indigenous therapeutics, Asian Journal of Counselling and Psychotherapy, 1(2), 111-124.

Bowers R., Plummer D. and Minichiello V. (2010) Religious attitudes, homophobia, and professional counselling, Journal of LGBT Issues in Counseling, 4(2), 70-91.

Bowers R. (2008) Counsellor Education as Humanist Colonialism – Pathways to an Indigenous Aesthetic, Australian Journal of Indigenous Education, 37, 71-79.

Bowers R. (2008) Reconnecting with the Mi'kmaq, Cape Breton University Mi'kmaq Resource Centre Online Publication, Sponsored by the University of New England, Armidale, NSW, Australia.

Bowers R. (2008a) Nukumij Tumaqn – Grandmother Medicine: Poetry from the Sacred Pipe, Cape Breton University Mi'kmaq Resource Centre Online Publication, Sponsored by the University of New England, Armidale, NSW, Australia.

Bowers R., Minichiello V. and Plummer D. (2007) Qualitative research in counselling: A reflection for novice counselor researchers, The Qualitative Report, 12(1), 131-145.

Bowers R. (2007a) A bibliography on Aboriginal and minority concerns: Identity, prejudice, marginalisation, and healing in relation to race, gender, sexuality, and the ecology of place, Counselling, Psychotherapy, and Health, 3(2), Indigenous Special Issue, 29-71.

Bowers R. (2007b) Clinical suggestions for honouring Indigenous identity for helpers, counsellors, and healers: The case of 'Marsha', Counselling, Psychotherapy, and Health, 3(2), Indigenous Special Issue, 13-28.

Bowers R. (2007c) Diversity in creation: Identity, race, sexuality and indigenous creativity, International Journal of Diversity in Organisations, Communities and Nations, 7(1), 3-7.

Bowers R. (2007d) Counsellor education as practice: An Australian narrative reflection on teaching and learning the practice of counselling in a university setting, Part Two, Counselling Australia, 7(1), 3-7.

Bowers R. (2006) Counsellor education as practice: An Australian narrative reflection on teaching and learning the practice of counselling in a university setting, Part One, Counselling Australia, 6(4), 8-11.

Bowers R. (2006a) Wholistic applications of counselling with the aging in dialogue with pastoral care concerns: A postmodern and transcendental analysis, Counselling, Psychotherapy, and Health, 2(1), 68-85.

Bowers R. (2005) Our stories, Our medicine – Exploring wholistic therapy integrating body-wellness, mindfulness, and spirituality: An Indigenous perspective on healing, change, and counselling, and the social and political contexts of an emerging discipline, Counselling Australia, 4(4)114-117.

Bowers R. (2005a) Shieldwolf and the shadow: Entering the place of transformation, Special Issue of the Australian Journal of Indigenous Education, Vol 34, 79-85.

Bowers R., Plummer D. and Minichiello V. (2005b) Homophobia in counselling practice, The International Journal for the Advancement of Counseling, 27(3), 471-489, September 2005.

Bowers R., Plummer D. and Minichiello V. (2005c) Homophobia and the everyday mechanisms of prejudice: Findings from a qualitative study, Counselling, Psychotherapy, and Health, 1(1) 31-57.

Bowers R. (2001) Life passages: Paths to empowerment for sexual minorities, Psychotherapy in Australia, 7(2), 60-66.

Brown, L. (Ed.) (1997). Two spirit people: American Indian lesbian and gay men, Haworth Park Press, New York.

Brown, L. (1997a) Women and men, not-men and not-women, lesbians and gays: American Indian gender style alternatives, In Brows L. (Ed.)., Two spirit people: American Indian lesbian women and gay men, Haworth Press, New York, 5-20.

Callender, C. & Kochems, L. (1983) The North American berdache (with comments and reply), Current Anthropology, 24(4), August-October, 443-470.

Champagne D. (1997) Preface: Sharing the gift of sacred being, In Brown L. (1997) Two spirit people: American Indian lesbian women and gay men, Haworth Press, New York, xvii-xxiv.

Chapple, M. and Kippax, S. (1996) Gay and homosexually active Aboriginal men in Sydney, National Centre in HIV Social Research School of Behavioural Sciences, Macquarie University, Melbourne, http://www.queers4reconciliation.wild.net.au/chapple.htm (1 November 2010).

Coleman, E. (2009) 'Toward Version 7 of the World Professional Association for Transgender Health's Standards of Care: Medical and Therapeutic Approaches to Treatment', International Journal of Transgenderism, 11: 4, 215 — 219.

Comeau M., Stewart S., Mushquash C. and Stevens D. (2005) New Developments among Mi'kmaq First Nations Youth, Paper presented at Issues of Substance Abuse, Canadian Centre on Substance Abuse National Conference 2005.

Cook S. (2005) Use of traditional Mi'kmaq medicine among patients at a First Nations community health centre, Canadian Journal of Rural Medicine, 10(2), 95-99.

Cornett C. (1995) Reclaiming the authentic self: Dynamic psychotherapy with gay men, Aronson, London.

Cortright, B. (1997). Psychotherapy and spirit: Theory and practice in transpersonal psychotherapy, State University of New York Press, New York.

Cowan J. (1992) Mysteries of The Dream-Time: The Spiritual Life of Australia Aborigines, Unity Press, Melbourne.

Cowan J. (1994) Myths of the dreaming: Interpreting aboriginal legends, Unity Press, Roseville.

Crocker K. (2005) The Dreamtime Narrative: Australian Aboriginal Women Writers, Oral Tradition and Personal Experience, www.arts.valberta.ca/cms/crocker.pdf , (9 November 2005).

Cruz L. (2014) Two Spirited Podcasts, Re:searching for LGBTQ Health, http://www.lgbtqhealth.ca/projects/two-spiritedpodcasts.php?ap=14#JeremyDutcher, (Accessed 13-8-17).

De Cecco J. (1990) Confusing the actor with the act: Muddled notions about homosexuality, Archives of Sexual Behavior, 19, 409-413.

Denzin N. and Lincoln Y. (2002) The Qualitative Inquiry Reader, Sage, San Francisco.

Denzin N. and Lincoln Y. (2003) Collecting and Interpreting Qualitative Materials, Sage, San Francisco.

Dorothy, L., Espelage, S., Swearer, M. (2008) Addressing Research Gaps in the Intersection Between Homophobia and Bullying, School Psychology Review, Bethesda: June, 37(2), 155-159.

Drazenovich G. (2015) Queer pedagogy in sex education, Canadian Journal of Education, 38(2)1-22.

Duran, E. & Duran, B. (1995) Native American postcolonial psychology, State University of New York, NY.

Duran, E. (2006) Healing the soul wound: Counseling with American Indians and other native peoples, Teachers College Press, Columbia University, NY.

Dutcher J. (2014) Two Spirited Podcasts, Re:searching for LGBTQ Health, http://www.lgbtqhealth.ca/projects/two-spiritedpodcasts.php?ap=14#JeremyDutcher, (Accessed 13-8-17).

Elm J., Lewis J., Walters K., Self J. (2016) 'I'm in this world for a reason': Resilience and recovery among American Indian and Alaska Native two-spirit women, Journal of Lesbian Studies, 20(3-4), 352-371.

Etter L., Moore C., McIntyre L., Rudderham S., and Wien F. (1999) The health of the Nova Scotia Mi'kmaq population: A final research report, Mi'kmaq Health Research Group.

Fekete J. (1987) Life after postmodernism: Essays on value and culture, St. Martin's Press, New York.

Ficova K. (2015) Two Spirit people and the LGBT community, Thesis for Bachelor of English Language and Literature, Department of English and American Studies, Masuryk University, Brno.

Foucault, M. (1978) The history of sexuality, Pantheon, New York.

Freire, P. (1978) Pedagogy of the Oppressed, Herder and Herder, NY.

Frontain R. (2003) Reclaiming the sacred: The bible in gay and lesbian culture, Harrington Park Press, New York.

Garrett, M., and Barret, B. (2003) Two spirit: Counseling native American gay, lesbian, and bisexual people, Journal of Multicultural Counseling and Development, April, 31(2), 131-142.

Gelso C., Fassinger R., Gomez M. and Latts M. (1995) Countertransference reactions to lesbian clients: The role of homophobia, counselor gender, and countertransference management', Journal of Counseling Psychology, 42(3), 356-364.

Giddens A. (1991) Modernity and self-identity: Self and society in the late modern age, Standford University Press, Standford.

Green, E. (1996) Rural youth suicide: The issue of male homosexuality. Social change in rural Australia, In Social change in rural Australia, Lawerence G. Lyons K. and Momtaz S. (Eds.), Rural Social and Economic Research Centre, University of Queesland, Rockhampton, 85-94.

Griffin D. (1988) Spirituality and society: Postmodern visions, State University of New York Press, New York.

Griffin G. (1998) Understanding heterosexism: The subtle continuum of homophobia, Women and Language, 21, 33-40.

Halberstam, J. (2005) Queer temporalities and postmodern geographies, In Halberstam, J. A queer time and place: Transgender bodies, subcultural lives, NY University Press, NY, 1-21.

Harris, J. (1990) One blood: Two hundred years of Aboriginal Encounter with Christianity: A Story of Hope, Albatross Books, Lion Publishing, London.

Harris P., Bartlett C., Marshall M., Marshall A. (2010) Mi'kmaq night sky stories: Patterns of interconnectiveness, vitality and nourishment, CAPjounral, 9(Oct)14-17.

Hatcher A., Bartlett C., Marshall M., Marshall A., Kavanagh S. (2010) Two-eyed seeing in the science classroom: Sampler of 'Two-Eyed Seeing' Curriculum for classroom teachers, Curriculum document, Cape Breton University, Sydney.

Herdt G. and Boxer A. (1993) Children of horizons: How gay and lesbian teens are leading a new way out of the closet, Beacon Press, Boston.

Holt N. (2003) Representation, legitimation, and auto ethnography: An auto ethnographic writing story, International Journal of Qualitative Methods, 2(1) Winter, 1-22.

Hornborg A-C. (2006) Visiting the six worlds: Shamanistic journeys in Canadian Mi'kmaq cosmology, Journal of American Folklore, Summer 2006, 312-336.

Hodge, D. (1993). Did you meet any malagas? A homosexual history of Australia's tropical capital, Little Gem Publications, Nightcliff.

Holmes-Whitehead R. (2002) Tracking Doctor Whiteshead: Showman to legend keeper – including the memoir of Jerry Lonecloud, Goose Lane Editions and Nova Scotia Museum, Halifax.

Holmes-Whitehead R. (1988) Stories from the six worlds: Micmac legends, Nimbus Publishing, Halifax.

Hunt S. (2016) An introduction to the health of Two-Spirit people: Historical, contemporary and emergent issues, National Collaborating Centre for Aboriginal Health, Prince George.

James C. and Shadd A. (1994) Talking about differences: Encounters in culture, language and identity, University of Toronto Press, Toronto.

Jones L. (2005) What Does Spirituality in Education Mean?: Stumbling Towards Wholeness, Journal of College & Character, 6(7), 1-7.

Kaufman G. and Raphael L. (1996) Coming out of shame: Transforming gay and lesbian lives, Doubleday, New York.

Knudtson P. and Suzuki D. (1992) Wisdom of the Elders, Stoddart Publishing, Toronto.

Krieger, C. (2002) Culture change in the making: Some examples of how a Catholic missionary changed Micmac religion, American Studies International, XL,2, June 2002, 37-56.

Lacey L. (1999) Medicine walk: Reconnecting with Mother Earth, Nimbus Publishing, Halifax.

Letendre A. (2002) Aboriginal traditional medicine: Where does it fit? Crossing Boundaries, 1(2), 78-87.

Levine, M. (2011) Lessons at the halfway point, Blackstone Audio, https://www.amazon.com/Lessons-Halfway-Point-Wisdom-Midlife/dp/1441784942 (Accessed 17-8-17).

Living Black (2009) Rainbow dreaming, http://news.sbs.com.au/livingblack/rainbow_dreaming_563593 (1 November 2010).

Marsden D. (2010) Creating and sustaining positive paths to health by restoring traditional-based Indigenous health-education practices, Canadian Journal of Native Education, 29(1), 135-146.

McIntyre L., Wien F., Rudderham S., Etter L. Moore C., MacDonald N., Johnson S., Gottschall A., (2001) An Exploration of the Stress Experience of Mi'kmaq On-Reserve Female Youth in Nova Scotia, http://www.acewh.dal.ca/eng/reports/ Wien%20Finalreport.pdf#search=%22M%C3%A9tis%20%22Mi'kmaq%22%20filetypeApdf%22, 22 August 2006.%4

Meads, C., Pennant, M., McManus, J. and Bayliss, S. (2009) A systematic review of lesbian, gay, bisexual and transgender health in the West Midlands region of the UK compared to published UK research, Unit of Public Health, Epidemiology & Biostatistics West Midlands Health Technology Assessment Group, The University of Birmingham.

Moore, Sr. Dorothy (2009) 'Teaching Mi'kmaw Students,' Social Justice Conference, 29 May 2009 [MG12,8 MRC 2013-8-4092 File#4 p.1, Sr. Dorothy Moore Papers, Mi'kmaq Resource Centre, Cape Breton University.

Morrow, R. & Brown, D. (1994) Critical theory and methodology: Contemporary social theory, volume 3, Sage Publications, New York.

MRC (2017) Mi'kmaq language, spirituality and medicine, https://www.cbu.ca/indigenous-affairs/unamaki-college/mikmaq-resource-centre/mikmaq-resource-guide/mikmaw-language-spirituality-medicine-mikmaw-tloti/, (Accessed 14-817).

Muncey T. (2005) Doing auto-ethnography, International Journal of Qualitative Methods, 4(1), 6-14.

Nadeau D. and Young A. (2006) Educating bodies for self-determination: A decolonizing strategy, Canadian Journal of Native Education, 29(1), 87-101.

Neu D. (2000) Accounting and accountability relations: Colonization, genocide and Canada's first nations, Accounting, Auditing & Accountability Journal, 13(3), 268-288.

Nakata, M. (2007) The cultural interface, The Australian Journal of Indigenous Education, 36S, 6-13.

National Indigenous Radio Service (2010) Dreaming 2010: Blaxxxuality in the 21st century, http://www.nirs.org.au/index.phpoption=com_content& view=article&id=4052:blaxxxuality&catid=27:the-dreaming&Itemid=143 (1 November 2010).

Nebelkopf , E. & Phillips, M. (Eds.). (2004) Healing and mental health for Native Americans: Speaking in red, Altamara Press, NY.

Noel L. (1994) Intolerance: A general survey, McGill Queen's University Press, Montreal.

Nova Scotia Government (2017) Mi'kmaw Community Gatherings, https://novascotia.ca/archives/mikmaq/resultsx.asp?Search=&SearchList1=2, (Accessed 14-817).

O'Neill C. and Ritter K. (1992) Coming out within: Stages of spiritual awakening for lesbians and gay men, Harper, San Francisco.

Orr, J. (2002) Decolonizing Mi'kmaw education through cultural practical knowledge, McGill Journal of Education, Fall 2002.

Orr, J. (2000) Learning from Native adult education, New Directions for Adult Education, 85(Spring), 59-66.

Outblack (2010) http://home.vicnet.net.au/~outblack/ what.htm (1 November 2010)

Paul, D. (2006) We were not the savages: Collision between European and Native American Civilizations, Fernwood Publishing, Halifax.

Peavy, R. (1993) Development of Aboriginal counselling: A brief submitted to the Royal Commission on Aboriginal Peoples, University of Victoria, http://www.bced.gov.bc.ca/abed/reports/subroyalcom.html, 26 July 2006.

Pereira, J. (2000) A Preliminary Case Study of Perceptions of Access to Ethnomedicine in the Environment in the Mi'kmaq Community of Indian Brook, http://www.collectionscanada.ca/obj/s4/f2/dsk1/tape4/PQDD_0016/MQ57222.pdf#search=%22M%C3%A9tis%20%20identity%20%22Mi%20Kmaq%22%20filetypeApdf%22, 22 August 2006.%4

Plummer, D. (2000) The quest for modern manhood: Masculine stereotypes, peer culture and the social significance of homophobia. Journal of Adolescence 23(1): 1-9. Available online at http://www.idealibrary.com.

Plummer D. (1999) One of the Boys: Masculinity, homophobia and modern manhood, Haworth Press, New York.

Razack S. (2007) What is to be gained by looking white people in the eye? Culture, race, and gender in cases of sexual violence, Feminism and the Law, 19(4), 894-923.

Restoule J-P. (2000) Aboriginal identity: The need for historical and contextual perspectives, Canadian Journal Education, 24(2), 102-112.

Robinson T. (1999) The intersections of dominant discourses across race, gender, and other identities, Journal of Counseling and Development, 77(Winter), 73-79.

Roscoe W. (1998) Changing ones: Third and fourth genders in Native North America, St Martin's Press, NY.

Roscoe W. (Ed.). (1988) Living the spirit: A gay American Indian anthology, St. Martin's Press, New York.

Said E. (1993) Culture and imperialism, Knopf, New York.

Sarup M. (1996) Identity, culture and the postmodern world, Edinburgh University Press, Edinburgh.

Schwanberg S. (1990) Attitudes towards homosexuality in American health care literature 1983-1987, Journal of Homosexuality, 19(3), 117-136.

Sedgwick, E. (1993) 'Epistemology of the closet' In The lesbian and gay studies reader, (Ed.), H. Abelove, M. Barale and D. Halperin, Routledge, New York.

Smith C. (2005) Epistemological intimacy: A move to auto ethnography, International Journal of Qualitative Methods, 4(2) June, 1-7.

Smith M. and Gordon R. (1998) Personal need for structure and attitudes toward homosexuality, The Journal of Social Psychology, 138(1), 83-88.

Sparrow C. (2006) Reclaiming spaces between: Coast Salish Two Spirit identities and experiences, Thesis for Master of Social Work, University of Victoria, Canada.

Stefanson S. (2009) Two Spirit sexuality in Native North American culture: Native Americans of alternative sexual orientations, http://www.suite101.com/content/indigenous-homosexuality-a2870 (Accessed 1 November 2010).

Stewart D. (2002) The role of faith in the development of an integrated identity: A qualitative study of black students at a white collage,' 43(4), 579-596.

St. Denis V. and Hampton E. (2002) Literature review on racism and the effects on Aboriginal education, http://www.sfu.ca/mpp/aboriginal/colloquium/pdf/Racism-and-Abo-Education.pdf, (27 March 2006).

St. Pierre, M. & Long Soldier, T. (1995) Walking in the sacred manner: Healers, dreamers, and Pipe Carriers – Medicine women of the Plains Indians, Simon & Schuster, NY.

Strelein L. (1998) This earth has an Aboriginal culture inside: Recognising the cultural value of country, Native Title Research Unit of the Australian Institute of Aboriginal and Torres Strait Islander Studies, Issues paper 23, 5-7.

Sylliboy J. (2017) Two-Spirits: Conceptualization in a L'nuwey Worldview, Thesis for Master of Arts Education, Mount Saint Vincent University, Halifax.

Tacey D. (2000) ReEnchantement: The New Australian Spirituality, Harper Collins Publishers, Sydney.

Taylor, C. (2008) Counterproductive Effects of Parental Consent in Research Involving LGBTTIQ Youth: International Research Ethics and a Study of a Transgender and Two-Spirit Community in Canada, Journal of LGBT Youth, 1936-1661, Volume 5, Issue 3, 2008, Pages 34 – 56.

Tompkins, J. (2002) Learning to see what they can't: Decolonising perspectives on Indigenous education in the racial context of rural Nova Scotia, McGill Journal of Education, 37(3), Fall, 405-422.

Tree, J. (2004) The way of the Sacred Pipe: The care and use of the Native American Sacred Pipe, Blue Sky Publishing, Hamilton.

Tucker N. (1995) Bisexual politics: Theories, queries, & visions, Harrington Park Press, New York.

Van-de-Ven, P., Bornholt, L. and Bailey, M. (1996) 'Measuring cognitive, affective, and behaviorial components of homophobic reaction' Archives of Sexual Behavior, 25(2), 155(125).

Walters, K., Evans-Campbell, T., Simoni, J., Ronquillo, T., and Bhuyan, R. (2006) 'My spirit in my heart': Identity experience and challenges among American Indian Two Spirit women, In Challenging lesbian norms: Intersex, transgender, intersectional, and queer perspectives, Harrington Park Press, NY, 125-150.

Walters, K., and Simoni, J. (2002) Reconceptualizing native women's health: A 'Indigenist' stress-coping model, American Journal of Public Health, 92(4), 520-524.

Walters, K., Evans-Campbell, T., Simoni, J., Horwath, P. (2001) Sexual orientation bias experiences and service needs of gay, lesbian, bisexual, transgender and two spirit American Indians, Journal of Gay and Lesbian Social Services, 13, 133-149.

Watt S. (1999) The story between the lines: The thematic discussion of the experience of racism, Journal of Counseling and Development, 77(Winter), 54-61.

Wells K. (2006) The origins of indigenism: Human rights and the politics of identity, Canadian Journal of Native Education, 29(2), 245-253.

Wesley D. (2015) Reimagining Two-Spirit community: Critically centering narratives of urban Two-Spirit youth, Thesis for Master of Arts, Queen's University, Kingston, Canada.

Wilber K. (1998) The marriage of sense and soul: Integrating science and religion, Random House, New York.

Wilber, K. (1995) Sex, Ecology, Spirituality: The Spirit of Evolution, Shambhala Press, NY.

Wilson, A. (1996) How we find ourselves: Identity development and two spirit people, Harvard Educational Review, 66(2), 303-317.

Woorama (2006) Indigenous homosexuality: Gay and transgender Aborigines and the colonization of sexuality, Yimpininni – Sistergirls, http://www.suite101.com/content/indigenous-homosexuality-a2870 (1 November 2010).

Young A. and Nadeau D. (2005) Decolonising the body: Restoring sacred vitality, Atlantis, 29(2), 1-13.

The Publisher

Ability Therapy Specialists Pty Ltd is a community-based project in counselling that assists individuals, families, and communities. We are a certified registered provider of the Australian National Disability Insurance Scheme and senior clinical members of the Australian Counselling Association. To learn more about our service please visit us at: www.abilitytherapyspecialists.com.au

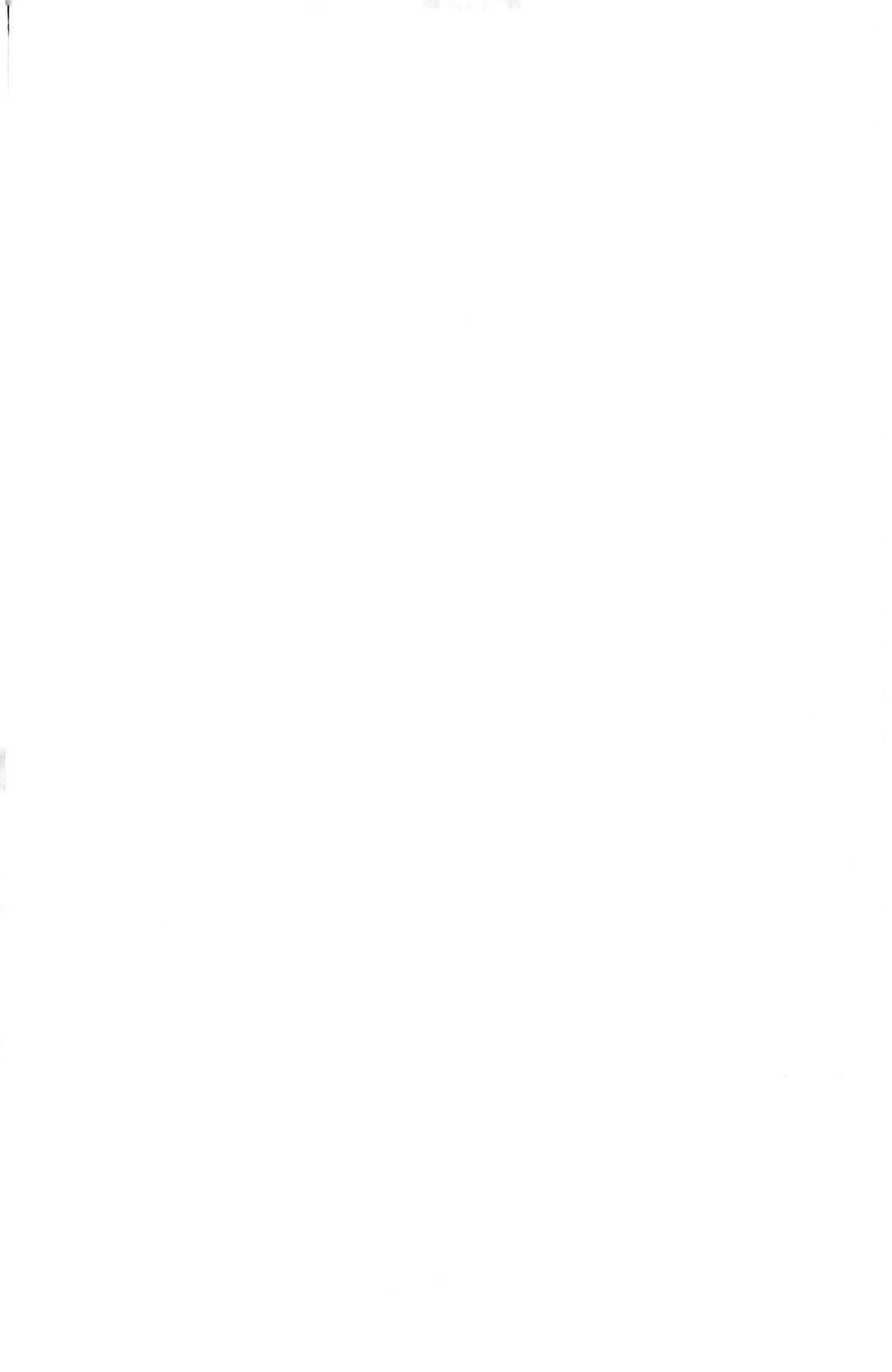

Manufactured by Amazon.ca
Bolton, ON